Evidence-Based
PHARMACOTHERAPY

OPTIMAL PATIENT CARE = BEST KNOWLEDGE + COMPETENT PRACTITIONER

Evidence-Based
PHARMACOTHERAPY

OPTIMAL PATIENT CARE = BEST KNOWLEDGE + COMPETENT PRACTITIONER

Elaine Chiquette and L. Michael Posey

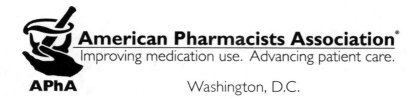

American Pharmacists Association®
Improving medication use. Advancing patient care.

APhA

Washington, D.C.

Acquiring Editor: Sandra J. Cannon
Managing Editor: Linda L. Young
Proofreader: Eileen Kramer
Compositor: Roy Barnhill
Cover Designer: Sarah Hoctor

© 2007 by the American Pharmacists Association

APhA was founded in 1852 as the American Pharmaceutical Association

Published by the American Pharmacists Association
1100 15th Street, N.W., Suite 400
Washington, D.C. 20005-1707
www.aphanet.org

To comment on this book via e-mail, send your message to the publisher at aphabooks@aphanet.org

Library of Congress Cataloging-in-Publication Data

Chiquette, Elaine.
  Evidence-based pharmacotherapy : optimal patient care=best knowledge +
competent practitioner / Elaine Chiquette and L. Michael Posey.
    p. ; cm.
  Includes bibliographical references.
  ISBN-13: 978-1-58212-068-3
  ISBN-10: 1-58212-068-4
  1. Chemotherapy. 2. Pharmacy. 3. Evidence-based medicine. I. Posey,
L. Michael. II. American Pharmacists Association. III. Title.
  [DNLM: 1. Drug Therapy. 2. Pharmacy. 3. Evidence-Based Medicine.
QV 704 C457e 2006]
  RM263.C49 2006
  615.5'8--dc22
                 2006100891

How to Order This Book

Online: www.pharmacist.com
By phone: 800-878-0729 (770-280-0085 outside the United States and Canada)
VISA®, MasterCard®, and American Express® cards accepted.

CONTENTS

FOREWORD

*A*T FIRST GLANCE, the concept of evidence-based pharmacotherapy would not seem particularly novel. We have always used evidence to make pharmacotherapeutic decisions. What might a book such as this one offer that is not already available in other books, texts, or references?

Although all clinicians make decisions involving drug therapy using the available evidence, the source of that evidence continues to evolve and change. The *evidence-based* approach represents a return to the empirical process of gathering information and a step away from—or beyond—the rational approach to choosing therapy that has been used in medical practice since the advent of the discipline of pharmacology less than 100 years ago.

This *empirical* approach to pharmacotherapy bases decisions on evidence gained from experience. Since the beginning of time, plant products and now synthetic drugs have been given to patients, the effects noted, and conclusions drawn. The difference today is in the methods—controlled clinical trials—used for evaluation of the effects. This approach does not require a theoretical lens through which to judge the effects, just a confidence in the power of the study methods.

In contrast, the *rational* approach to pharmacotherapy requires a theoretical basis for making decisions, starting with an understanding of the pathophysiology of disease and then developing pharmacologic approaches to alter the disease. This rational construction follows in the footsteps of other theories used to understand disease and formulate drug therapy decisions. The theory of the four humors—blood, black bile, yellow bile, and phlegm—was the rational construct used to explain disease from the time of Hippocrates until just over 100 years ago. Chiropractic, osteopathy, naturopathy, and other theories also were developed to provide a rational basis for curing disease.

Classic pharmacology, originating in Germany in the early part of the 20th century, is a rational approach derived from a strict mechanistic view of the world: If one can develop a new drug molecule that jiggles a receptor, ties up an enzyme, or binds a biologic constituent, then the drug should produce changes in the human body that lead to prevention or cure of disease or amelioration of its symptoms.

The evidence-based approach to the care of people represents a return to this type of rational, empirical approach. Its only requirement is that decisions be based on an orderly evaluation of what actually happens in other people as the basis for predicting what will happen in the patient at hand. This approach is no different than the experience-based approach used by medicine men, curanderos, grannywomen, root doctors, herbalists, and other folk healers throughout history.

What is different, however, are the methods used to evaluate this experience. Strict scientific processes—the randomized clinical trial, the prospective cohort, or case–control study—have been developed to assure us that we are "seeing" a pattern of response that truly is there.

Evidence-Based Pharmacotherapy explains techniques for evaluating these scientific methods, along with methods of finding and applying this new type of evidence. This text moves in an orderly fashion, starting with a thorough explanation of what an evidence-based approach to pharmacotherapy entails. Chapters follow on finding and evaluating this information, understanding the results of the research, and applying the evidence. The editors have performed a great service by collecting the various tools of evidence-based pharmacotherapy and placing them on an enclosed compact disc.

Evidence-Based Pharmacotherapy represents what I hope will be the start of a movement in pharmacotherapy away from an approach limited by a tenacious adherence to theory. While we cannot abandon the basic sciences of medicine, since they form the base on which to build an evidence-based approach, we have to realize that their usefulness is limited in the care of real people with real health problems. We have to embrace the idea that patients do not "read the book" and that drug therapy that is *supposed* to work may not do so. While not rejecting these rational underpinnings, we have to embrace the idea that experience, well measured, trumps theory.

This book will show you how.

Allen F. Shaughnessy, PharmD, BCPS, FCCP
Tufts University Family Medicine Residency
Boston, Massachusetts

December 2006

PREFACE

*T*HREE YEARS AGO, when this book was just a dream consisting of a few notes in a word-processing file, medication-related problems had already been recognized as the cause of much unnecessary morbidity and mortality among patients around the world. Beginning in the mid-1990s, studies were demonstrating that for every dollar spent on medications, at least another dollar was spent on medical care for resulting drug-related problems or on the productivity lost to society when patients were unable to work or had died of adverse drug effects.

Today, the problem is recognized as being at least that bad and probably worse, especially for a graying population whose frail elderly are taking multiple medications for multiple chronic diseases. Yet, even as the Medicare Part D program, which was another dream until December 2003, recognizes the need for medication therapy management services for these senior citizens, everyone remains preoccupied with the costs of the drugs themselves, failing to appreciate how important it is to manage that drug therapy, empower patients to become partners in their own care, and emphasize that patients make the right lifestyle choices when they are younger that can provide healthier lives as they age.

Evidence-Based Pharmacotherapy is dedicated to the proposition that optimal patient care is delivered by competent practitioners who have access to the best knowledge that medical research can provide. As the dominant modality of care in the health care system of the early 21st century, pharmacotherapy is key to the prevention and treatment of human disease, and the health professional who is able to access, interpret, and apply the best evidence concerning the use of medications will ensure optimal outcomes for his or her patients.

This book is intended to serve as both an introductory textbook for students learning about the connection between research and practice, and as a useful guide to pharmacists and other health professionals who are seeking to incorporate evidence-based medicine into their use of medications in treatment or prevention of disease. In a succinct, easy-to-read format, we have worked to create a roadmap for clinicians to follow in applying the best studies in the burgeoning clinical literature to the care of patients—one at a time.

Beginning with an introduction to evidence-based pharmacotherapy in Chapter 1, the book takes students and readers through the steps of a sound decision-making process. Chapter 2, "Searching the Biomedical Literature: Finding a Needle in a Haystack," helps the busy clinician formulate a drug information question and learn how to use the clinical literature to find an answer relevant for a given patient. The reader is introduced to different computer-based information sources and provided with validated search strategies.

Chapter 3 takes the next step by showing readers the importance of "Matching the Question With the Best Available Evidence." Here we distinguish between strong and weak evidence and describe the process of detailed critical appraisal. The relative strengths of several types of evidence sources are reviewed, including randomized controlled trials, observational designs, practice guidelines, and systematic reviews.

The numbers attached to study findings have stumped many a clinician, so in Chapter 4, Gilbert Ramirez, DrPH, of the Charles R. Drew University of Medicine and Science in Los Angeles, shares his secrets on "Demystifying Statistics." He provides basic information about descriptive and inferential statistics with a focus on the appropriate use and interpretation of statistical tests. This chapter also covers how different displays of information (e.g., standard deviation versus standard error of the mean, Y-axis scale) may distort the results and confuse the interpretation of results.

In clinical practice, the ultimate question is whether the potential benefits or harm described in a study are clinically important for an individual. Chapter 5 offers tools to (1) find the best clinically relevant outcome; (2) translate the results into meaningful numbers that assess the magnitude of the effect; and (3) incorporate clinical expertise, resources, and patient preferences, and values before moving to action.

The basic principles of decision analysis are presented in Chapter 6, "Making a Pharmacotherapy Decision Using a Decision-Analytic Framework." In this chapter, Matthew Sarnes, PharmD, of Xcenda in Princeton, New Jersey, focuses on structuring the decision-making process to ensure that the most appropriate course of action is chosen and optimal outcomes therefore ensured.

Since an increasing number of health care decisions are influenced or made outright at the corporate level, Chapter 7 presents information on "Applying Evidence-Based Pharmacotherapy to Formulary Decisions." Written by Sheri Ann Strite and Michael Stuart, MD, of the Defini Group, LLC, in Portland, Oregon, and Seattle, Washington, respectively, this chapter provides insights into how evidence-based practice is used in making the decisions reached by formulary and pharmacy & therapeutics committees. Specifically, it explains (1) what a formulary system is; (2) the advantages and disadvantages of using a formulary system; (3) the qualities of an effective system, including details about an evidence- and value-based approach; (4) how to conduct scientific, clinical and economic drug reviews; and (5) how to effectively—and efficiently—use various resources available to ensure high quality of the information used to support formulary decisions.

The book closes with the reminder that the final answer is never known. "Keeping Up to Date" provides lifelong learning tools to help clinicians stay current and organized. These tools include reference manager software that can facilitate filing and retrieval systems by creating a virtual library, "current awareness" services, which send e-mail alerts when new evidence of interest to the user is published, handheld downloads to access data at the point of care, and interview techniques to get the most from visits by pharmaceutical company field representatives.

In addition to these chapters, the textbook includes a compact disc with useful, computer-based, supplemental information and exercises that will test the skills learned in several chapters.

We take this opportunity to thank our colleagues in APhA's Books and Electronic Products Department, Julian Graubart, Sandy Cannon, and Kathy Anderson; our editor and project manager, Linda Young; Dawn A. Cox for assistance with tables and graphics; Josée Ricard, BPharm, MSc, for sharing with us some of the drug information requests received at du Centre d'information sur le médicament at Laval University; Cindy Mulrow, MD, for sharing with us both directly and through her many publications what evidence-based medicine means; and those colleagues—especially Scott Richardson, MD, and Bill Linn, PharmD—who have influenced us in the evidence-based pharmacotherapy realm over the years. Without the support and encouragement of these people, we would have lacked the insights and drive to push this dream through to fruition.

Elaine Chiquette, PharmD
San Antonio, Texas

L. Michael Posey, BPharm
Athens, Georgia

December 2006

CONTRIBUTORS

Elaine Chiquette, PharmD
Senior Medical Science Liaison
Amylin, Medical Affairs
San Antonio, Texas

L. Michael Posey, BPharm
Editorial Director, Periodicals
Editor, *JAPhA, Pharmacy Today*, and *APhA DrugInfoLine*
Pharmacy Editor, Books and Electronic Products
American Pharmacists Association
Athens, Georgia

Gilbert Ramirez, DrPH
Program Director and Professor
Master in Urban Public Health
College of Science and Health
Charles R. Drew University of Medicine and Science
Los Angeles, California

Matthew Sarnes, PharmD
Senior Director
Xcenda
Princeton, New Jersey

Sheri Ann Strite
Principal & Managing
Partner
Delfini Group, LLC
Portland, Oregon

Michael Stuart, MD
President
Delfini Group, LLC
Seattle, Washington

INTRODUCTION TO EVIDENCE-BASED PHARMACOTHERAPY

L. Michael Posey and Elaine Chiquette

∽
Scenario
∽

Ms. NM is a 44-year-old mother of two, a 17-year-old girl and a 12-year-old boy. She was diagnosed 3 years ago with breast cancer. The tumors were removed surgically, and she underwent a recommended course of chemotherapy. She has since been taking tamoxifen as part of a planned 5-year adjuvant regimen.

Recently, clinical evidence increasingly supports the use of aromatase inhibitors, rather than tamoxifen, for this adjuvant care. After reading a newspaper article that described a study on letrozole (Femara— Novartis) published in the New England Journal of Medicine *and hearing that the Food and Drug Administration had approved the drug as first-line adjuvant care, Ms. NM approaches her pharmacist and asks whether she should talk with her oncologist about changing her medication.*

WHEN IT COMES TO HELPING PATIENTS reach important decisions about their bodies and the interventions that will be applied to them, health professionals provide a tremendous service when they translate their years of education and experience into a recommended course of action for an individual person. What is the best way for health professionals to do this? Where do pharmacotherapists, medication therapy managers, and other clinicians get the information on which they base their recommendations? How do they mesh the cold, hard data of large clinical trials with what they observe day in and day out in their own practices? How can they be sure they are coming to sound conclusions without being unduly influenced by marketing hype or the hope that a new therapy is a miracle cure?

We believe this book will help health professionals address those hard questions. Increasingly, medicine and society in general are coming to one conclusion when it comes to health professionals' recommendations: If not evidence based, what? Patients are free to accept or reject evidence-based recommendations (as evidenced by the boom in use of dietary supplements, many of which have little evidence to support their effectiveness or safety). But health professionals are held to this standard when it comes to explaining, rationalizing, and, in some cases, defending their advice.

In this textbook, the basic principles of evidence-based medicine (EBM) will be described as they apply in the unique world of pharmacotherapy, with the emphasis on balancing benefits and harms of medications and formulary debates. (Appendix 1–A provides a glossary of common terms used in EBM.) The steps pharmacists can take in making evidence-based analyses are also presented, along with strategies for staying up to date and continuously incorporating new findings into their daily practice.

Becoming Interpreters of Drug Information

～
Scenario
～

Mr. WM, husband of Ms. NM, is a 49-year-old executive in the banking industry. His sedentary, high-stress job has taken a toll on his body over the years; he currently is obese and a smoker, and drinks three to four alcoholic beverages a day. In the years since his wife was diagnosed with breast cancer, his blood pressure has increased and is reaching the threshold that requires treatment, his blood glucose levels place him in the prediabetic range, and his lipids are elevated.

At his annual physical examination, Mr. WM hears his physician describe the likely clinical course of someone in this situation. The doctor notes that, on the basis of the Framingham study, a large longitudinal research effort [see http://www.framingham.com/heart], Mr. WM has a 15% chance of a major cardiovascular event during the next 10 years.

The apothecary in olden times and more recently "Doc" in the corner drugstore played an important role in people's lives. While today's pharmacists may not always have the close personal relationship that was possible in less complex societies of the past, the impact of prescription screening, counseling, education, advice, and encouragement go far beyond what many patients today comprehend.

Pharmacists evolved during the 20th century from purveyors of individually compounded medicaments to dispensers of manufactured dosage forms, and then to clinical pharmacists, pharmacotherapists, and providers of pharmaceutical care.[1-4] With this evolution came new responsibilities, ones that must be supported by the same pillars that provide the structure, the processes, and ultimately the value of medicine. As stated by Hepler and Strand[5] in their definition of pharmaceutical care, these elements are as follows:

> Pharmaceutical care involves the process through which a pharmacist cooperates with a patient and other professionals in designing, implementing, and monitoring a therapeutic plan that will produce specific therapeutic outcomes for the patient. This in turn involves three major functions: (1) identifying potential and actual drug-related problems; (2) resolving actual drug-related problems; and (3) preventing potential drug-related problems.

Building on the foundation of the clinical pharmacy movement of the 1960s, pharmacists in the 1990s and the 2000 decade have now transformed this concept of pharmaceutical care into the medication therapy management services that are covered under the Medicare Part D benefit implemented at the beginning of 2006.[6] In a wide variety of practice settings, pharmacists have proven that the application of their unique knowledge of drugs and diseases can be applied to the benefit of the patient. Pharmacists' accessibility and ability to coach and communicate have benefited patient care and improved outcomes in the tens of thousands of community pharmacies, hospitals, ambulatory care clinics, nursing homes and other long-term care facilities, and managed care organizations.[7]

The bottom line is that pharmacists are well-educated—and well-paid—members of the health care team who have the responsibility to provide information to the rest of the team and pharmaceutical care to the patient. To meet this weighty challenge, pharmacists need to know the best ways of improving medication use and advancing patient care. To do so—to interpret information about medications accurately and perceptively—pharmacists need to apply the principles of EBM, that is, to practice evidence-based pharmacotherapy.

History of Evidence-Based Medicine

∾
Scenario
∾

Mr. WM's father, now in his early 70s, was recently diagnosed with mild Alzheimer disease, and the family is contemplating moving him into a nursing home that specializes in the care of patients with this progressive disease. Mr. WM has been reading up on the condition, and he believes that drug treatment with one of the cholinesterase inhibitors should be started now. While visiting the nursing home, he asks to speak with the consultant pharmacist, and he presses her on why the home is not using more of these medications for patients in early stages of the disease.

The move toward emphasizing the quality of clinical evidence can be traced to the 19th century,[8] but the modern seed that became EBM was planted in 1972 with publication of the book *Effectiveness and Efficiency: Random Reflections on Health Services*, written by Professor Archie Cochrane, an epidemiologist in Scotland.[9] He wrote that obstetric and other health practices were flawed because its practitioners were failing to incorporate findings of randomized controlled trials into daily decisions and recommendations. Cochrane also argued that systematic reviews were needed to provide overall summaries of clinical trials, which were beginning to increase in number and quality.

Murray Enkin and his colleagues[10] at Oxford University took up Cochrane's challenge, culminating in the late 1980s with publication of the book *A Guide to Effective Care in Pregnancy and Childbirth*. On the other side of the Atlantic, David Sackett and colleagues at McMaster University developed the concept of EBM further, and Sackett was later appointed director of the newly founded Centre for Evidence-Based Medicine in Oxford, England. The Cochrane Collaboration was founded in 1993; since then thousands of monographs have been posted to provide evidence-based summaries of knowledge in dozens of clinical areas.[11]

Making the Move Toward Evidence-Based Practice

∾
Scenario
∾

Ms. NM's younger sister and her 3-year-old daughter come to stay with the family during the winter holidays. The little girl develops otitis media for which a local pediatrician prescribes a 5-day course of amoxicillin. When the prescription is presented to Ms. NM's pharmacist, she calls the pediatrician to question both the decision to treat the otitis media, given the equivocal clinical results obtained in clinical trials, and, if antibiotics are to be used, the decision to use a 5-day course.

Pharmacists are perfectly positioned in the prescribing process to detect and resolve errors and suboptimal medication choices; they also generally like and agree with the principles of EBM.[12] But pharmacists' impact has been limited by their lack of access to patients' health information.

As technologic innovations, such as the availability of health information on Web-based systems or on cards that patients might carry, become realities, this barrier will be eliminated, and pharmacists will be able to apply fully their years of education and experience.

In anticipation of pharmacists providing a new level of pharmaceutical care and medication therapy management, colleges of pharmacy have increasingly moved toward case-based learning and other approaches to teaching student pharmacists how to use their knowledge in making clinical decisions and recommendations. However, requiring that students apply the principles of EBM has not been a consistent universal emphasis in this process. Medical schools made this shift many years ago,[13] and the authors and others[14] believe that the time is now for a renewed emphasis on evidence-based pharmacotherapy in both pharmacy school curricula, continuing education programs and certificate courses, and the pharmacy literature.

The Bottom Line

> Pharmacists are increasingly becoming the purveyors of interpreted drug information that other professionals and patients use in making important treatment decisions.
> EBM evolved in the latter half of the 20th century to become the standard of care in clinical medicine.
> Pharmacists and student pharmacists should incorporate evidence-based pharmacotherapy into their daily recommendations to other health professionals and patients, and use its principles in building drug formularies.

References

1. Kusserow RP. The Inspector General's report on the clinical role of the community pharmacist. Washington, D.C.: U.S. Government Printing Office; 1990.

2. ACCP Clinical Practice Affairs Committee. Clinical pharmacy practice in the noninstitutional setting: a white paper from the American College of Clinical Pharmacy. *Pharmacotherapy*. 1992;12:358–64.

3. Bluml BM, McKenney JM, Cziraky MJ. Pharmaceutical care services and results in Project ImPACT: hyperlipidemia. *J Am Pharm Assoc*. 2000;40:157–65.

4. Cranor CW, Christensen DB. Short-term outcomes of a community pharmacy diabetes care program: the Asheville project. *J Am Pharm Assoc*. 2003;43:149–59.

5. Hepler CD, Strand LM. Opportunities and responsibilities in pharmaceutical care. *Am J Pharm Educ*. 1989;53:7S–15S.

6. American Pharmacists Association and National Association of Chain Drug Stores Foundation. Medication therapy management in community pharmacy practice: core elements of an MTM service (version 1.0). *J Am Pharm Assoc*. 2005;45:573–9.

7. Posey LM. Proving that pharmaceutical care makes a difference in community pharmacy. *J Am Pharm Assoc*. 2003;43:136–9.

8. Sackett DL, Rosenberg WMC, Muir Gray JA, et al. Evidence based medicine: what it is and what it isn't [editorial]. *BMJ*. 1996;312:71–2.

9. Cochrane AL. *Effectiveness and Efficiency: Random Reflections on Health Services*. London: Nuffield Provincial Hospitals Trust; 1972. [Reprinted in 1989 in association with the *BMJ*. Reprinted in 1999 for Nuffield Trust by the Royal Society of Medicine Press, London (ISBN 1-85315-394-X).]

10. Enkin M, Keirse MJNC, Chalmers I. *A Guide to Effective Care in Pregnancy and Childbirth*. Oxford: Oxford Medical Publications; 1989.

11. Starr M, Chalmers I. The evolution of The Cochrane Library, 1988–2003. Available at http://www.update-software.com/history/clibhist.htm. Accessed: October 6, 2006.

12. Burkiewicz JS, Zgarrick DP. Evidence-based practice by pharmacists: utilization and barriers. *Ann Pharmacother.* 2005;39:1214–9.

13. Evidence-Based Medicine Working Group. Evidence-based medicine. A new approach to teaching the practice of medicine. *JAMA.* 1992;268:2420–5.

14. Matowe L. Evidence-based medicine—is pharmacy keeping up? *Pharm J.* 2000;265:893.

APPENDIX 1-A

GLOSSARY OF EVIDENCE-BASED MEDICAL TERMS*

Terms to Describe Benefit or Harm of Treatment

	Outcome	
Exposure	**Event**	**No Event**
Treated (experimental group)	a	b
Control (unexposed group)	c	d

Experimental event rate (EER): The proportion of patients in the treated group in whom an event is observed. Thus, if out of 100 treated patients ($a+b$), the event is observed in 27 (a), the event rate is 0.27 ($a/a+b$).

Control event rate (CER): The proportion of patients in the control group in whom an event is observed. CER = $c/c+d$.

Absolute risk: The risk of having a disease at any point in time (incidence). For example, if the incidence of a disease is 1 in 100,000, then the absolute risk is 0.001%.

Absolute risk reduction (ARR): The difference in the event rate between control group (CER) and treated group (EER): ARR = CER – EER.

Number needed to treat (NNT): The inverse of the ARR (1/absolute risk reduction). NNT is the number of patients who need to be treated to prevent one bad outcome. If a drug reduced the risk of a bad outcome (e.g., stroke, myocardial infarction, death) from 40% to 20%, then:

ARR = 0.2 (EER [event rate in the experimental/treatment group])
   – 0.4 (CER [event rate in the control group])|
   = |0.4 – 0.2 | = 0.2 (20%)

So,

NNT = 1/ARR
   = 1/0.2 = 5

Thus, five people would need to be treated with the drug to prevent one bad outcome.

Relative risk (RR): A ratio of two risks, the risk of the outcome/event in the treated group compared with the risk of the outcome in those not exposed (control group). This value is also referred to as *risk ratio*. Reported as a percentage, it is calculated as RR = EER/CER. A relative risk above 1 means the treatment/exposure is associated with the outcome, and a value below 1 means the treatment is negatively associated with the outcome.

---

* Editor's Note: Glossary terms reproduced from Dipiro JT, Talbert RL, Yee GC, et al. *Pharmacotherapy: A Pathophysiologic Approach.* 5th ed. New York: McGraw-Hill; 2002. Adapted with the permission of The McGraw-Hill Companies. Copyright 2002.

Relative risk reduction (RRR): The proportional reduction in events between control and treated groups. Reported as a percentage, it is calculated as (CER – EER)/CER or as 1 – RR.

Absolute risk increase (ARI): The risk difference in outcome rates between treated and control groups when the treatment harms more patients than the control. ARI is calculated as EER – CER.

Number needed to harm (NNH): The inverse of ARI (1/absolute risk increase). NNH is the number of patients who would need to be treated to cause one adverse outcome.

Odds ratio (OR): A ratio that describes the odds (probability) that a patient in an exposed or intervention group had an event (usually harmful event) relative to the odds that a patient in the control group had that event. When the outcome of interest is rare, the odds ratio approximates the relative risk. Odds ratio is used·in case–control or retrospective trials. It is calculated as OR = odds of being exposed in cases (*a/c*) divided by odds of being exposed in controls (*b/d*).

Terms to Describe Study Designs

Blinded study: Study in which neither the study subject nor the study staff knows to which group or intervention the subject has been assigned in a double-blinded study. In a single-blinded study, only the subject is not aware of his or her assignment. Blinding minimizes bias.

Case–control study: Retrospective comparison of causal factors or exposures in a group of persons with disease (cases) and those of persons without the disease (controls). The purpose is to find the clinical finding that occurs more frequently in the cases than in the control. The relative risk is estimated by the odds ratio (OR).

Case series: Report on a series of patients with a specific disease. No control group is included.

Cohort study: Retrospective or prospective follow-up study of exposed and nonexposed defined groups in which a variable of interest, usually disease rates, is measured. Exposure is measured before development of disease. Incidence, risk, and relative risk are measured.

Crossover study: A trial comparing two or more treatments in which the participants, on completion of the course of one treatment, are switched to another. The therapies are administered in either a specified or random order to each participant.

Cross-sectional study: A study that examines the presence or absence of a disease and other variable in a defined population, and the potential risk factors at a particular point in time or time interval. Exposure and outcome are determined simultaneously. The temporal sequence of cause and effect cannot necessarily be determined.

Meta-analysis: A systematic review that uses quantitative methods to summarize the results. The unit of analysis in the meta-analysis, rather than the patient, is the variable common to the studies being reviewed.

Open-label trial: A study in which the investigators assign the interventions rather than using random allocation, and both patients and investigators know which patients are receiving which therapies or interventions.

Randomized controlled trial: A comparative study in which the researchers randomly assign patients to treatment or control groups. Random allocation means that each participant has the same chance of receiving each of the possible groups under investigation.

Systematic review: A comprehensive summary of best available evidence that addresses a defined question. The study uses systematic and explicit methods to identify, select, and critically appraise and collect data from relevant research. Systematic reviews may or may not include a quantitative analysis (such as that used in meta-analysis).

SEARCHING THE BIOMEDICAL LITERATURE: FINDING A NEEDLE IN A HAYSTACK

Elaine Chiquette

*F*ORMULATING A QUESTION AND SEARCHING FOR RELEVANT INFORMATION are the first two steps in the process of making an evidence-based recommendation about clinical care of a patient. Clinicians today face a virtual cacophony of information, with e-mail and Web sites promising coverage of breaking medical news in addition to the insights offered by textbooks and by articles, reviews, and meta-analyses in biomedical journals, which have exploded in number over the past half century.

In this chapter, the process of effectively formulating an accurate question is presented along with descriptions of how the biomedical literature can be searched effectively for relevant information about questions related to evidence-based medicine.

Identifying Background Versus Foreground Questions

Background Questions

Most questions that pharmacists encounter in daily practice are background questions. They relate to common, well-known, or well-studied issues. There are two elements to the background question: (1) a question root: who, what, where, how, or why and (2) the drug or disorder/disease, as illustrated in the following examples:

1. Who makes Viagra?
2. What is the active ingredient in Sudafed PE?
3. Why was fenfluramine removed from the market?
4. How do I make metformin syrup?
5. Why can't I give gentamicin and ampicillin together in the same line?
6. Where can I administer insulin (abdomen, arm, or thighs)?

Examples of resources that will help answer background questions include textbooks, handbooks, reference texts, databases, review articles, and Web sites. The best source of the information, however, is a secondary resource, that is, a resource that condenses and summarizes evidence derived from original studies. (For example, a review article published in the journal

Pharmacotherapy is a secondary source; the textbook *Pharmacotherapy: A Pathophysiologic Approach* is a tertiary source.) Original studies are referred to as primary sources because they describe results of authors' original research. Using a secondary resource is much more time efficient compared with reading original articles. The advantages of secondary resources are that they cover a broad topic, are a great source for background information, are usually readily available to pharmacists, and provide references that can be retrieved for more details if needed. A disadvantage is that they may be out-of-date.[1]

Foreground Questions

Foreground questions ask specific knowledge about patient management. These questions require processing several elements simultaneously (the effect of the intervention considering the patient's condition, the standard management, and the outcome of interest). The following section dissects the components of a foreground question.

Formulating a Focused Question

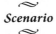

Scenario

The emergency room nurse calls you at the pharmacy asking whether enoxaparin (Lovenox—sanofi-aventis) can be used intravenously.

As you investigate further, the nurse explains that a 57-year-old man presented in the emergency room with an acute myocardial infarction, and Dr. MI has prescribed enoxaparin 30 mg iv followed by 1 mg/kg sc. The nurse explains that she looked in the package insert and found nothing about using the drug intravenously. Is this use safe?

Creating a Searchable Question

As illustrated in the user tip and Figure 2–1, there are four elements to a well-formulated question: the patients or problem being addressed, the intervention being considered, the comparison groups or gold standard, and the outcome(s) of interest.[2]

User Tip

The acronym PICO is a useful aide-mémoire:

P = Patient or problem: Who is the patient? Describe the specific patient population.
I = Intervention: What is the drug regimen? Define the therapy (dose, frequency, route, length) or procedure.
C = Comparison: What is the alternative? Is it better or worse than what? A gold standard? No treatment? Or placebo?
O = Outcome: What is the effect of the intervention?

A PICO feature is available on the main screen of PubMed (http://pubmedhh.nlm.nih.gov), and uses a fill-in-the-blank and menu format to help in searches for information.

User Tip (continued)

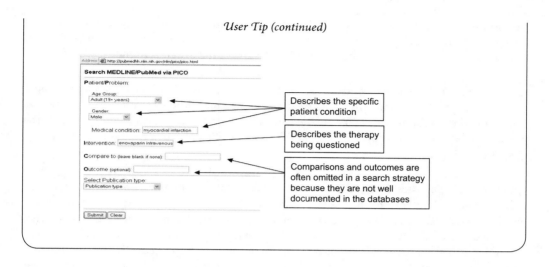

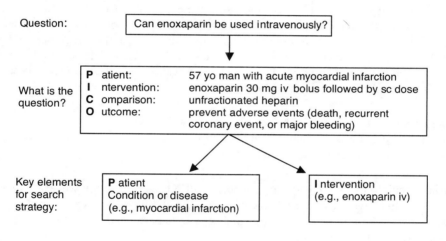

Figure 2–1

Elements of a well-formulated searchable clinical question. iv = intravenous; sc = subcutaneous.

Patient or Problem The most common patient descriptor is the disease itself. The question posed in the scenario does not relate to an orthopedic patient receiving enoxaparin for thromboprophylaxis or a patient newly diagnosed with deep vein thrombosis, but rather to a patient presenting with an acute myocardial infarction. Other useful components to describe the patient of interest include age, ethnicity, gender, pregnancy, renal and liver function, concomitant medications, and past medical history. For example, whether the patient is older than 75 years or has impaired renal function may significantly change the answer about the safety of using enoxaparin.

Intervention   In this case, the pharmacist is being asked about a low-molecular-weight heparin, more specifically enoxaparin used intravenously at a 30 mg fixed dose followed by a subcutaneous weight-based dose. The question relates to giving the drug intravenously.

Comparison   This step involves defining the treatment against which the intervention should be compared. If a gold standard exists such as unfractionated heparin for acute myocardial infarction, the gold standard should be the comparison for efficacy or safety questions. Or the nurse may really want to know whether intravenous use of enoxaparin is as safe as enoxaparin given subcutaneously.

Outcome   The last step is to define the efficacy and safety outcomes. In this scenario, the safety outcome of interest to the nurse is assumed to be bleeding or, more specifically, major bleeding events. Other examples of safety outcomes include death, teratogenicity, and renal impairment. Efficacy outcomes refer to improved symptoms, survival, or decreased morbidity. For practical reasons, efficacy most commonly refers to improved surrogate markers of survival or cure. Surrogate markers or intermediate outcomes are risk factors, predictors that cannot be felt by patients but are associated with morbidity or mortality outcomes.[3] For example, blood pressure is a surrogate outcome; it cannot be felt by patients, but is associated with adverse health outcomes such as stroke and death. Patients cannot feel an increase in low-density lipoprotein cholesterol, C-reactive protein, adenomatous colonic polyps, decreased bone mineral density, or abnormal glycosylated hemoglobin, but each of these surrogate end points is associated with morbidity or mortality outcomes. (This article provides more information on surrogate endpoints: Fleming TR, DeMets DL. Surrogate endpoints in clinical trials: Are we being misled? *Ann Intern Med.* 1996:125;605–13.)

A Generic Searchable Question   The generic format of the PICO process can be expressed as follows: In this <u>P</u>atient, is the <u>I</u>ntervention better, worse, or equivalent to the <u>C</u>omparison to prevent or improve the <u>O</u>utcome of interest?

Scenario-Specific Searchable Question   The specific PICO question for this scenario is expressed as follows: In this 57-year-old man with acute myocardial infarction, is enoxaparin 30 mg iv followed by 1 mg/kg sc better than unfractionated heparin to prevent adverse events (major bleeding, death, recurrent coronary event)?

Searching the Best Source

Faced with a question, the pharmacist has a limited number of options to try to identify the best answer to both types of questions:

1. Ask an expert colleague
2. Review a textbook
3. Consult an electronic database of systematic reviews
4. Conduct a literature search using an electronic database of primary literature
5. Search the World Wide Web

The pharmacist should consider the advantages and disadvantages of each of these options.

Ask a Colleague

 ➤ Easy, inexpensive, and quick
 ➤ Favored for background questions

A colleague with more experience can be a great source of answers to background questions. He or she has been exposed to background questions several times already, has researched them, has formulated answers, and is willing to share the information. This strategy is good for commonly known information or questions unique to the person's professional experience (e.g., compounding a recipe, total parenteral nutrition mix, IV compatibility of medications), but caution is warranted if the question relates to medications commercialized more than 5 years after a colleague graduated because the person's knowledge may not be up-to-date.[4] The volume and complexity of medical information are growing exponentially, making the task of keeping up to date very difficult for everyone.

Review a Textbook

 ➤ Choose the textbook carefully
 ➤ Favored for background questions

A textbook is as good as its authors. Clinicians should carefully review author qualifications and remember that authors will have biases based on their own experience. Whether the text is based on expert opinion or evidence is important. Important questions to consider in selecting a textbook are what process was used to update the textbook and when was it last updated?

The survival kit for pharmacists to answer background questions should include a representative textbook in each of the following 10 categories (Table 2–1 presents selected lists of useful textbooks in each category):

1. Drug monographs
2. Drug interactions
3. Adverse drug reactions
4. Drug dosing in special population (renal or liver impairment, pregnancy, lactation, pediatrics, geriatrics)
5. Drug identification (foreign or not)
6. Toxicology (treatment of poisoning)
7. Nonprescription drugs (including complementary and alternative medicines)
8. Drug compounding
9. Stability and compatibility of drugs
10. Clinical medicine

Consult Electronic Databases of Systematic Reviews

 ➤ Systematically summarizes all and only the best evidence
 ➤ Favored for foreground questions

A *systematic review* is a review that strives comprehensively to identify and synthesize all literature on a given topic. The unit of analysis is the primary study, and the same scientific principles and rigor apply as for any study. If a review does not state clearly whether and how all relevant studies were identified and how the information from them was synthesized, it is not a systematic review.

Table 2-1 Background Question/Tertiary Resources

	S	Format	Price*	Web Address or Contact Information	Description
General Compounding					
Professional Compounding Centers of America (PCCA)	Y	W		http://www.pccarx.com 1-800-331-2498	PCCA provides compounding technical support, training, and sourcing for hard-to-find chemicals.
International Academy of Compounding Pharmacists	Y	L	300.00 (Int); 500.00 (U.S.)*	http://www.iacprx.org	An international, nonprofit association that protects and promotes the art and skill of pharmaceutical compounding.
Trissel's *Stability of Compounded Formulations*	N	T	92.00	http://www.pharmacist.com	Provides a single compilation of all currently available stability information on drugs in compounded oral, internal, topical, and ophthalmic formulations.
International Journal of Pharmaceutical Compounding	Y	W/J	150.00 (R) 180.00 (I)*	http://www.ijpc.com	*IJPC* is a bimonthly, scientific, and professional journal emphasizing quality pharmaceutical compounding, which features hands-on and how-to compounding techniques.
Pharmacy Times Compounding Page	N	W/J	Free	http://www.pharmacytimes.com	Compounding hotline is a repository of questions and answers related to compounding. Information is limited, but users can e-mail questions to Mr. Erickson.
Drug Identification					
Ident-A-Drug	Y	W/T	39.00	http://www.identadrug.com	Identifies drug products by the codes imprinted on them as well as by the color and shape of the product.
The Pharmaceutical Journal	Y	W	Free for identification of most drugs	http://www.pharmj.com	Internet site can be accessed free of charge. The links are electronic resources to help identify foreign drugs.
Martindale: The Complete Drug Reference	Y	T/W/D	†	http://www.micromedex. com/products/martindale	Contains information on drugs in clinical use worldwide. Also available as a database within Micromedex Healthcare Series.

Name		Format	Cost	URL	Description
Identidex	Y	W	†	http://www.micromedex.com/products/identidex	Database available within Micromedex Healthcare Series. Identifies tablets and capsules by imprint code and secondary characteristics such as color and shape.
Index Nominum	Y	W	†	Within Micromedex	Database available within Micromedex Healthcare Series. Is an international drug directory providing access to more than 5300 substances and derivatives, more than 12,800 synonyms, and more than 41,800 trade names from more than 45 countries.
Toxicology					
Poisondex	Y	W	†	http://www.micromedex.com	Micromedex Healthcare Series database. Resource to help identify and treat accidental or intentional exposures; provides information on clinical effects, range of toxicity, and treatment protocols.
Lexi-Comp: Poisoning & Toxicology	Y	W/T/PDA	399.00 online; 75.00 PDA	http://www.lexi.com	This database provides information on drugs, chemical agents, and environmental toxins, and appropriate tests and treatments for each substance.
American Association of Poison Control Centers	N	W	Free	http://www.aapcc.org 1-800-222-1222	Provides information on potential poisoning medications and emergencies.
Drug Interactions					
Drugs.com	N	W	Free	http://www.drugs.com	Provides comprehensive and up-to-date drug information online.
Drug-Reax System	Y	W/T	†	http://www.micromedex.com	Provides drug–drug, food–drug, drug–disease, drug–ethanol, drug–tobacco, drug–alternative medicine, and drug–laboratory assay interactions.
Medscape	Y	W	Free	http://www.medscape.com/druginfo	Provides drug–drug interaction information via their drug database or the multidrug interaction checker. Information can be printed for the patient.
Natural Products					
Natural Medicines Comprehensive Database	Y	W/T	92.00	http://www.naturaldatabase.com	Evidence-based resource provides information, including reactions, on herbal medicines and dietary supplements.

Table 2-1 (continued) Background Question/Tertiary Resources

	S	Format	Price*	Web Address or Contact Information	Description
AltMedDex (Micromedex database)	Y	W/T	†	http://www.micromedex.com	This database offers evidence-based, clinical information on herbal, vitamin, mineral, and other dietary supplements. The unbiased information is peer reviewed by a team of experts from both alternative medicine and traditional medicine communities. Editorial board members performing the reviews include physicians, pharmacists, nurses, and naturopathic doctor.
Adverse Drug Reactions					
Micromedex	Y	W/T	†	http://www.micromedex.com	Micromedex can answer clinical questions by providing trusted medical information and by combining evidence-based content with flexible technology.
Clin-Alert	Y	T	120.00	http://cla.sagepub.com/	A quick reference to adverse clinical events.
AHFS Drug Information	Y	W/T	215.00*	http://www.ashp.org	Provides drug information, interactions, and drug monographs.
eFacts	Y	W/D	459.95*	http://www.factsandcomparisons.com	Provides one-click access to details about drug interaction facts.
Mosby's Drug Consult	Y	W/T	59.95	http://www.mosbysdrugconsult.com	Provides prescribing information for thousands of complete generic entries, as well as cost of therapy, product identification, international brand names, patient information, Orange Book equivalents, method of supply, and average wholesale price.
MedWatch	N	W	Free	http://www.fda.gov/medwatch/	Internet gateway for safety information on the drugs and other medical products regulated by the U.S. FDA.
Meyler's Side Effects of Drugs	Y	T	426.00	http://www.arsmedica.com	A worldwide yearly survey of new data and trends in adverse drug reactions, published every 4 years.
Special Populations (Pregnancy, Renal, Pediatric)					
ReproRisk (available as a database within Micromedex)	Y	T/W	†	http://www.micromedex.com/products/reprorisk/	Databases to help in evaluating human reproductive risks of drugs, chemical, and physical/environmental agents.

Name				URL	Description
Harriet Lane Handbook	N	T/PDA	49.95	http://www.us.elsevierhealth.com/	Pediatrics textbook with downloadable PDA.
Drugs in Pregnancy and Lactation, 7th Edition	N	T/PDA	99.00	http://www.lww.com/	Provides information on fetal and neonatal risks to drugs and biologicals.
Nephrology Pharmacy Associates	Y	W/J	Free	http://www.nephrologypharmacy.com	Committed to applying its nephrology pharmacy expertise to improve quality and delivery of health care to renal patients.
Patient Information					
MedlinePlus	N	W	Free	http://www.nlm.nih.gov/medlineplus/druginformation.html	Provides free printable information, in PDFs.
DrugDigest	N	W	Free	http://www.drugdigest.org	Provides comprehensive reviews of drugs, easy-to-use drug interaction tool, drug comparison tool (side-by-side comparison of drugs in the same class). DrugDigest is the consumer health and drug information Web site of Express Scripts, Inc., the nation's largest independent pharmacy benefit manager.
Nonprescription Drug Products					
Handbook of Nonprescription Drugs, 15th Edition	N	T/PDF	$144	http://www.otchandbook.com/	Used as a textbook in many schools of pharmacy, this APhA publication provides a clinical perspective on the diseases and conditions most commonly treated with nonprescription medications. Includes information on therapeutic choices, criteria for when patients should be referred for medical care, and complementary and alternative medicines.
eFacts	Y	W/D	459.95*	http://www.factsandcomparisons.com/	
Micromedex	Y	W/T	†	http://www.micromedex.com/	Provides clinical solutions to help improve patient outcomes, reduce medication errors, and streamline management of diseases/conditions.
Physicians' Desk Reference (PDR)	Y	W/T/D	92.00-99.95	http://www.pdr.net/login/Login.aspx	The drug information on *PDRhealth* is written in lay terms and is based on the FDA-approved drug information found in the PDR.

Table 2-1 (*continued*) Background Question/Tertiary Resources

	S	Format	Price*	Web Address or Contact Information	Description
Disease Management Resource					
UpToDate	Y	W/D	495.00*	http://www.uptodate.com/	An electronic, full-text clinical resource that provides instantaneous, evidence-based answers to the most commonly asked questions in clinical practice. Specialities covered in depth by UpToDate include adult primary care, cardiology, family practice, gynecology, infectious diseases, oncology, and women's health. Original material in UpToDate is written by an international faculty of practicing clinicians who are experts in their specialties.
MD Consult	Y	W/D	199.95*	http://www.mdconsult.com/	Includes almost 40 renowned medical texts, articles from more than 50 clinical journals, over 600 practice guidelines, drug information, 2500 patient education handouts, CME, and daily medical updates.
Stat!Ref	Y	W	65.00	http://www.statref.com/	Stat!Ref Electronic Medical Library provides quick access to a number of full-text medical reference books covering the areas of diagnosis and treatment in a variety of medical specialties, such as psychiatry, geriatrics, obstetrics and gynecology, cardiology, and surgery. Texts on coding, drug information, and abbreviations and acronyms are also available.
Harrison's Principles of Internal Medicine	Y	W/T	135.00	http://harrisons.accessmedicine.com/	Harrison's Online is the online version of *Harrison's Principles of Internal Medicine*, one of the world's leading medicine textbooks. Updated daily.

	S		$	Description	URL
Compatibility					
Trissel's *Tables of Physical Compatibility*	Y	W/T	499.00	Provides physical compatibility information and drug stability for use in a clinical setting.	http://www.trissels.net/
King Guide to Parenteral Admixtures	Y	W/T/D	240.00	Complete intravenous drug reference available in CD-ROM and PDA formats.	http://www.kingguide.com/
IV Index (available within Micromedex)	Y	W	†	Searches two main databases: Trissel's Tables and Gold Standard Multimedia® - IV Admixture Information.	http://www.micromedex.com/
Drug Price					
Mosby's Drug Consult	Y	W/T	59.95	Provides drug information and prices.	http://www.mosbysdrugconsult.com/
Red Book	N	T	99.00	Provides latest pricing and product information on more than 100,000 Rx and OTC items. Also includes a broad spectrum of health care information.	http://www.pdrbookstore.com/
Clinical Calculators					
New York Emergency Room RN	N	W	Free	Developed for nurses in training. Has comprehensive list of medical formulas.	http://www.geocities.com/nyerrn/z/pda.htm
MedCalc 3000	Y	W	29.00	Comprehensive list of medical formulas. Has a pocket PC version. Also includes diagnostic criteria and treatment algorithms.	http://medcalc3000.com/

S = Subscription required; $ = price for subscription/product in U.S. dollars as of 2006; Y = yes; W = Web site; L = letter; T = textbook; J = journal; Int = international pharmacist; U.S. = U.S. pharmacist; R = regular price; I = institutional price; D = CD-ROM; N = no; PDA = personal digital assistant.

* Price may be lower for student pharmacists: Micromedex Healthcare Series prices vary depending on pharmacy school involvement (free to student pharmacists if school is registered) and/or package bundle.

† Micromedex Healthcare Series prices also vary depending on hospital size

Consulting electronic databases of systematic reviews and meta-analyses limits the amount of time health care professionals have to research and review the literature before they answer clinical questions or reach patient care decisions. Busy health care professionals prefer summaries of information. Traditional narrative reviews are useful for broad overviews of particular therapies of diseases or for reports on the latest advances in a particular area for which research may be limited.[5] However, information from narrative reviews is often gathered ad hoc, and the author's bias may enter into the process of gathering, analyzing, and reporting information.

In contrast, systematic reviews employ a comprehensive, reproducible data search and selection process to summarize all the best evidence. Systematic reviews follow a rigorous process to appraise and analyze the information, quantitatively (through the meta-analysis technique) or qualitatively, to best answer a defined clinical question. These reviews are a useful means of assessing whether findings from multiple individual studies are consistent and can be generalized.[6] The Centre for Reviews and Dissemination has created several strategies to identify meta-analyses from MEDLINE. The strategies can be found at http://www.york.ac.uk/inst/crd/search.htm.

⌒ Scenario ⌒

You receive a call at the pharmacy from a pregnant woman who wishes to buy a cream to prevent stretch marks. She asks you whether anything has been studied. You have access to your local university library and decide to search the Cochrane Library. You find a systematic review "Creams for preventing stretch marks in pregnancy" by Young and Jewell. The authors report that, compared with placebo, treatment with a cream containing Centella asiatica extract, alpha-tocopherol, and collagen–elastin hydrolysates appears to help prevent the development of stretch marks in women who have previously suffered stretch marks in pregnancy.

The Cochrane Library

The Cochrane Library is a relatively new and growing electronic library that provides more than 1000 systematic reviews of randomized controlled trials about the efficacy and safety of pharmaceutical and other interventions to improve health (see http://www.cochrane.org for further details). The library adds new summaries four times a year to its cumulative online and CD-ROM versions. With new reviews being added with each issue of the Cochrane Library, all areas of health care eventually will be covered.

The library is the product of a grassroots network, the Cochrane Collaboration, which began in 1993. This international nonprofit organization represents a worldwide network of more than 4000 health care professionals, researchers, and consumers working together toward a similar goal: to prepare, maintain, and disseminate systematic reviews of the effects of health care.

Creating a Cochrane review involves the systematic assembly, critical appraisal, and synthesis of all relevant studies that address a specific clinical question. Reviewers use strategies that limit bias and random error. These strategies include a comprehensive search for potentially relevant articles and selection of specific articles, using explicit, reproducible criteria. Reviewers critically appraise research designs and study characteristics during synthesis and interpretation of results. When appropriate, they integrate the results using meta-analysis. The unique value of Cochrane reviews is the commitment to regular updating. Reviews published in journals are often out-of-date by the time they are published. By updating reviews as new evidence becomes available, the Cochrane Library provides the current best evidence for health care decision makers.

The Cochrane Database of Systematic Reviews is the key component of the Cochrane Library, but not its only jewel. The library has three other databases: Cochrane Controlled Trials Registry, Database of Abstracts of Reviews of Effectiveness, and the Cochrane Review Methodology Register. The Database of Abstracts of Reviews of Effectiveness (DARE) is produced by the United Kingdom National Health Services Centre for Reviews and Dissemination, and contains citations to thousands of systematic reviews that were prescreened for quality. The Cochrane Controlled Trials Registry is a collection of citations of randomized controlled trials identified by using MEDLINE searches, hand searches of journals not indexed by MEDLINE, and other sources of randomized controlled trials. The Cochrane Review Methodology Database is a bibliography of journal articles and books addressing methodologic issues relevant to conducting a systematic review. (The section Centre for Reviews and Dissemination provides further information about these databases.)

PubMed/MEDLINE now index the Cochrane reviews. If a university subscribes to Ovid, students can also search the two main Cochrane databases (DARE, Cochrane Review Methodology Register). Figure 2–2 illustrates the search for a Cochrane review on stretch marks using the Cochrane Database of Systematic Reviews within PubMed.

An alternative to using the limit "Review" is to type the word "Cochrane" within the search box (Figure 2–3). PubMed will search for this word within all fields (including the database field [i.e., Cochrane Database of Systematic Reviews]), as shown in Figure 2–4.

The Cochrane reviews follow a structured format to help the reader browse through the review. Specific to a review are (1) synopsis: a summary specifically developed with the non–health care professional in mind, (2) details about the selection criteria of trials included in the systematic review, (3) tables summarizing the methodologic qualities of each trial included, and (4) conclusions subdivided by the impact of the review on practice and the impact on future research.

The table in Figure 2–4 is pulled from the Cochrane review of "creams for preventing stretch marks in pregnancy." Included in this table is one study of pregnant women reporting the efficacy of a cream (N = 41) to prevent the development of striae gravidum compared with placebo (N = 39). At the end of the trial, women who received the cream were less likely to develop stretch marks, compared with those who received placebo (odds ratio, 0.41; 95% CI, 0.17–0.99).

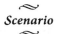

Scenario

You participate as a member of an institution's pharmacy and therapeutics (P&T) committee. You are charged with the task to review pioglitazone (Actos—Takeda Pharmaceuticals North America, Inc.) and rosiglitazone (Avandia—GlaxoSmithKline) for type 2 diabetes and make a recommendation back to the committee about which agent should be preferred.

National Institute for Clinical Excellence Database

The National Institute for Health and Clinical Excellence (NICE) is part of the United Kingdom National Health Service; its main responsibility is to perform clinical and economic reviews of drugs and devices to make recommendations for a national formulary. The database provides systematic reviews of technologies and drug therapies to health care professionals. NICE's technology appraisal is very comprehensive and often includes nonpublished information provided in confidence by the manufacturer. Throughout the appraisal process, NICE follows the Cochrane methodology to develop reviews.

Step 1.

Step 2.

Step 3.

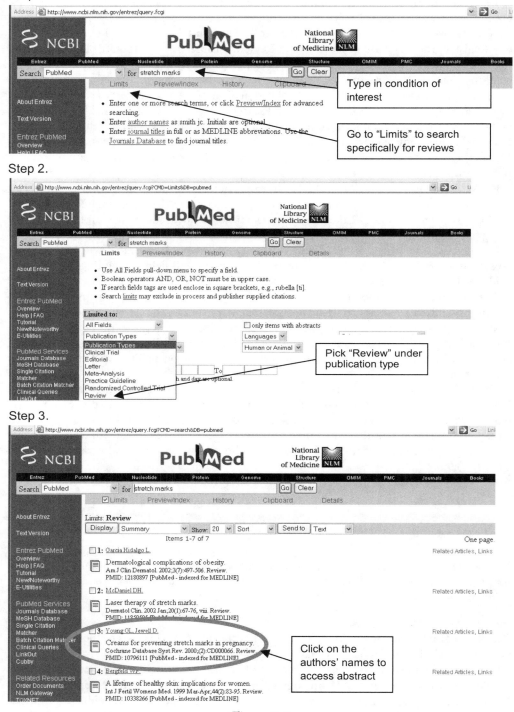

Figure 2–2

Search of Cochrane reviews using PubMed search box.

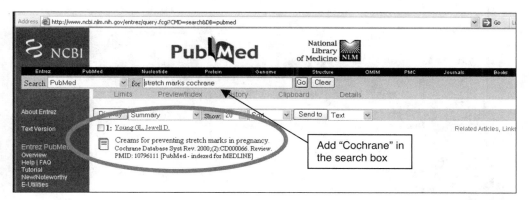

Figure 2-3
PubMed search for Cochrane reviews using the term "Cochrane" in the search box.

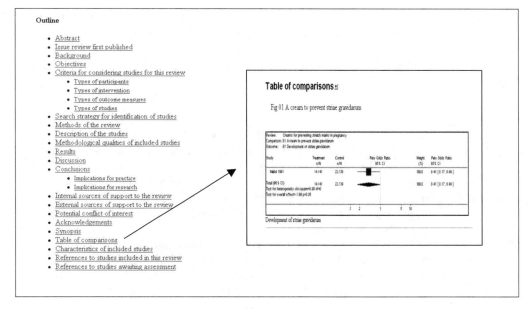

Figure 2-4
Example of a table of results in a Cochrane review. Young GL, Jewell D. Creams for preventing stretch marks in pregnancy. Cochrane Database of Systematic Reviews: Reviews 1996 Issue 1 John Wiley & Sons, Ltd Chichester, UK DOI: 10.1002/14651858.CD000066. (Copyright Cochrane Collaboration, reproduced with permission.)

The NICE Web site (Figure 2–5) has a health technology report for pioglitazone and one for rosiglitazone, along with a summary of the organization's recommendations about the use of thiazolidinediones for diabetes. The full technology report is more than 140 pages and includes meta-analyses for several outcomes such as the effect of thiazolidinediones on glycosylated hemoglobin, blood pressure, and lipids. The disadvantage of NICE technology reports is that they are not always up-to-date, but they certainly offer a great start for a P&T review.

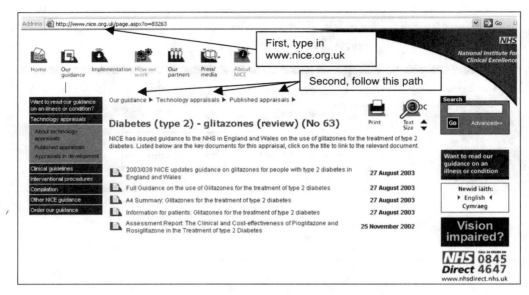

Figure 2–5

The NICE database. (National Institute for Health and Clinical Excellence [NICE] [2006], www.nice.org. uk, reproduced with permission.)

Centre for Reviews and Dissemination

The Centre for Reviews and Dissemination (CRD) was established in January 1994 in the United Kingdom. It aims to provide quality information about the effects of interventions used in health and social care. The CRD systematically screens several databases (e.g., MEDLINE, EMBASE, Cochrane) to identify quality reviews (systematic reviews and meta-analyses) on the clinical and economic impact of health care interventions. The CRD has three main databases. DARE contains more than 2500 structured abstracts of good quality published reviews about the effectiveness of health interventions. The NHS [National Health Service] Economic Evaluation Database (NHS EED) is a repository of abstracts summarizing good quality economic evaluation of drugs and devices. The Health Technology Assessment (HTA) database includes the work from the International Network of Agencies for Health Technology Assessment. All databases also can be accessed free on the Internet at http://www.york.ac.uk/inst/crd. Searching for "pioglitazone" or "rosiglitazone" will return 19 and 20 hits, respectively (as of October 2006), from which information can be chosen for the P&T report. The search provided the link to a NICE health technology report for pioglitazone and rosiglitazone, and also found an economic evaluation published in the journal *PharmacoEconomics,* a Cochrane review, and a Canadian technology report.

Refer to Evidence-Based Clinical Guidelines

As their names suggest, evidence-based clinical guidelines are guided by objective data and should be preferred over guidelines based on expert opinion that refer loosely to evidence to support their opinions. Expert-opinion guidelines vary in their scientific validity and reproducibility.[7]

The National Guideline Clearinghouse's Web site provides links to many evidence-based clinical practice guidelines. For each guideline, this comprehensive database offers a short summary of the key attributes, including the bibliographic sources, guideline developers and endorsers, status of the guidelines, and major recommendations. Recently added to the Web site is the ability to download the recommendation to a handheld device for easier access at the point of care. Table 2–2 presents an annotated list of additional resources for evidence-based clinical practice guidelines.

Table 2-2 North American Sources of Evidence-Based Clinical Practice Guidelines

Resource Description	Special Features
National Guideline Clearinghouse (NGC) (http://www.guideline.gov) NGC is a collaboration of U.S. Department of Health and Human Services, Agency for Healthcare Research and Quality (AHRQ), in partnership with the American Medical Association (AMA) and the American Association of Health Plans (AAHP). NGC provides access to full-text guidelines (when available) produced by a number of different professional medical associations and health care organizations. Each guideline is critically appraised with the use of a standard instrument. The site permits comparison of several guidelines side by side.	➣ Approx. 500 guideline summaries ➣ Weekly e-mail alerts ➣ Advanced search queries based on guideline attributes ➣ Annotated bibliography of resources relevant to guideline methodology ➣ Downloadable on Palm OS
National Library of Medicine's Health Services/Technology Assessment Text (http://www.ncbi.nlm.nih.gov/books/bv.fcgi?rid=hstat) This Internet resource is a collection of AHRQ-supported guidelines, AHRQ technology assessments and reviews, ATIS (HIV/AIDS Technical Information), NIH Warren G. Magnuson clinical research studies, NIH Consensus Development Program, Public Health Service (PHS) Guide to Clinical Preventive Services, and the Substance Abuse and Mental Health Services Administration's Center for Substance Abuse Treatment.	➣ Hundreds of full-text guidelines ➣ Metasearch capabilities to PubMed, the Centers for Disease Control and Prevention (CDC) Guidelines Database and the National Guideline Clearinghouse ➣ Access to quick-reference guides for clinicians and consumer brochures
Primary Care Clinical Practice Guidelines (http://medicine.ucsf.edu/resources/guidelines) This Internet resource offers a listing of online guidelines. The site is searchable by clinical content and organization.	➣ Guidelines and clinical reviews ➣ Cross-cultural health ➣ Teaching, patient information, and more ➣ Users' Guides to the Medical Literature - Rational Clinical Exam
CDC Prevention Guidelines Database (http://wonder.cdc.gov/wonder/prevguid/prevguid.html) This site is a comprehensive collection of all the official CDC guidelines and recommendations for prevention of diseases, injuries, and disabilities.	➣ More than 500 prevention guidelines/ documents ➣ Searchable ➣ Sorted by date, topic, or alphabetical order
Cancer Care Ontario Practice Guidelines Initiative (CCOPGI) (http://hiru.mcmaster.ca/ccopgi/guidelines.html) This Web page includes published and unpublished guidelines related to cancer care. These guidelines are created by the CCOPGI and are available as full text.	➣ Approx. 45 guidelines ➣ When information is scarce, evidence summary is created to review the best evidence available

Table 2-2 (continued)   North American Sources of Evidence-Based Clinical Practice Guidelines

Resource Description	Special Features
Clinical Practice Guidelines and Protocols in British Columbia (http://www.hlth.gov.bc.ca/msp/protoguides/gps/index.html) The guidelines and protocols are developed under the direction of an advisory committee and follow a rigorous review process. Guidelines are evaluated every 2 years for updates.	➤ Approx. 55 guidelines ➤ Patient guide also included for most guidelines
Clinical Practice Guidelines Infobase (http://www.cma.ca/cpgs/index.asp) Guidelines in this collection were produced or endorsed in Canada by a national, provincial, or territorial medical/health organization, professional society, government agency, or expert panel. The database is searchable by category, title, or developer. Full text is provided when available.	➤ Approx. 255 guidelines ➤ More than 2000 documents (reviews in both French and English) ➤ Advanced search capabilities
The Agency for Healthcare Research and Quality Evidence-Based Practice Centers (AHRQ EPCs) (http://www.ahcpr.gov/clinic/epcix.htm) AHRQ has established 12 EPCs to analyze and synthesize the scientific literature, and develop evidence reports and technology assessments on clinical topics.	➤ More than 100 evidence reports ➤ Full text available
The Ontario Guideline Advisory Committee (GAC) (http://gacguidelines.ca) The GAC assesses the rigor and clinical relevance of existing clinical practice guidelines and recommends the best source on the basis of their critical appraisal.	➤ More than 60 guidelines critically appraised and summarized

Source: Chiquette E, Posey LM. Evidence-based medicine. In: *Pharmacotherapy: A Pathophysiologic Approach.* DiPiro JT, Talbert RL, Yee GC, et al. New York: McGraw-Hill; 2005:29. Adapted with permission of The McGraw-Hill Companies. Copyright 2005.

Conduct a Literature Search Using Electronic Databases

Dozens of electronic databases exist as primary sources of original research reports (Table 2-3). MEDLINE and PubMed, produced by the National Library of Medicine (NLM), are the best-known bibliographic databases of biomedical journal literature. Although the MEDLINE database began in 1966, the NLM is also indexing retrospectively and creating a database called OldMEDLINE that dates back to 1953. Another NLM database, PreMEDLINE, contains the citations to articles that are "in-process" for MEDLINE, but not yet completely indexed. These citations can be searched by using text words, even though the subject headings have not been added. Several interfaces/platforms exist to access the MEDLINE database (e.g., FirstSearch, Ovid, PubMed, and SilverPlatter WebSPIRS). PubMed has some major advantages over the other platforms: It is free, the only platform that includes both OldMEDLINE and PreMED-LINE citations, and usually the platform in which new articles are listed first. However, the search capabilities in PubMed, although much improved, are still not as sensitive as other platforms.

Table 2-3 Electronic Bibliographic Databases

Electronic Database	Description
Alt-Health Watch (http://www.epnet.com/eptech)	Contains full text of periodicals, peer-reviewed journals, academic and professional publications, magazines, consumer newsletters and newspapers, research reports, and association newsletters focused on complementary, alternative, and integrated approaches to health care and wellness.
AMED (Allied and Alternative Medicine) (http://www.amed.org.uk)	Contains citations* from more than 350 biomedical journals covering the fields of complementary or alternative medicine and allied health. The database includes English-language and European sources; newspapers and books are also indexed.
ARTEMISA (Articulos Editados en Mexico Sobre Informacion en Salud)	Contains medical and pharmaceutical citations, and is considered the premier medical database in Mexico.
Biological Abstracts (http://www.biosis.org/products/ba)(Also available through Ovid)	Contains references to life science journal literature from 1972 to the present. Coverage is international, and includes agriculture, biochemistry, biomedicine, biotechnology, botany, ecology, microbiology, pharmacology, and zoology.
CAM Citation Index (http://nccam.nih.gov)	Contains approximately 180,000 bibliographic records on published CAM research over the last 35 years. Available through the NCCAM (National Center for Complementary and Alternative Medicine) Web site.
CINAHL (Cumulative Index to Nursing and Allied Health Literature) (http://www.cinahl.com) (Also available through Ovid)	Contains information about ongoing internal and commissioned projects that is most relevant to nursing care.
Cochrane Controlled Trial Registry (http://www.cochrane.org) (Also available through Ovid within the evidence-based medicine databases)	Contains references of randomized controlled trials and systematic reviews identified from electronic bibliographic sources and hand searching of multiple journals.
CRISP (Computer Retrieval of Information on Scientific Projects) (http://crisp.cit.nih.gov)	Contains information about research supported by the U.S. Public Health Service.
ExtraMED (http://www.iwsp.org/extraMED.htm)	Contains references of approximately 300 journals from developing countries.
EMBASE (http://www.embase.com)	Contains biomedical and pharmaceutical citations, and is considered the premier biomedical database in Europe.
HealthSTAR (Health Services, Technology, Administration, and Research) (http://www.nlm.nih.gov/pubs/techbull/mj99/mj99_healthstar.html)	Contains citations to published literature in health services, technology, administration, and research.
IBIDS (International Bibliographic Information on Dietary Supplements) (http://ods.od.nih.gov/Health_Information/IBIDS.aspx)	Contains citations published in international scientific journals on the topic of dietary supplements including vitamins, minerals, selected herbal, and botanical supplements from 1986 to the present.

Table 2–3 (continued)   Electronic Bibliographic Databases

Electronic Database	Description
IBIS (Integrative Body Mind Information System) (http://www.ibismedical.com)	Contains more than 250 reviews of the impact of complementary medicine for common medical conditions. It references standard textbook and authoritative sources in the complementary medicine field.
LILAC (Literature Latino Americana y del Caribe en Ciencia de al Salud)	Contains citations to medical literature that are published in Latin America and the Caribbean (Spanish literature).
MEDLINE (http://www.pubmed.org) (Free database available through PubMed and Ovid)	Indexes almost 4600 international biomedical journals from 1966 to the present. Includes references from Index Medicus, International Nursing Index, and Index to Dental Literature, and is considered the premier biomedical database in the United States. Also includes Cochrane reviews.
Napralert (http://www.napralert.org)	Napralert contains bibliographic data on 100,000 natural compounds and covers pharmacology, biological activity, and chemistry. It requires special access and searching expertise.
NHS CRD HTA (National Health Service Centre for Reviews and Dissemination, Health Technology Assessment)	Contains abstracts produced by International Network of Agencies for Health Technology Assessment and other health care technology agencies.
PsychLIT (http://www.apa.org/psycinfo)	PsychLIT is a computerized CD-ROM database produced by PsychINFO. It provides access to the international journal, book-chapter, and book literature in psychology. The database covers more than 1300 journals in 27 languages from approximately 50 countries.
Rosenthal Center for Complementary and Alternative Medicine (http://www.rosenthal.hs.columbia.edu/Botanicals.html)	Contains 56 searchable electronic databases (Aerzte Zetung, Acupuncture Literature Analysis and Retrieval System, Phytodoc, etc.; no subscription required).
ToxLine (http://toxnet.nlm.nih.gov/)	Contains online bibliographic information covering the biochemical, pharmacologic, physiologic, and toxicologic effects of drugs and other chemicals (no subscription required).

Note: Bibliographic databases are time efficient, relatively inexpensive, and widely available. They require some experience to use their search tools, and have inconsistent coding and variable indexing.

* Citations include information about the article such as the authors' names, the article title, the journal it is published in, the page numbers, year of publication, and usually an abstract.

MEDLINE includes citations from nearly 4000 leading biomedical journals.[8] The citations are not full-text articles, rather each citation includes authors' names, article title, journal name, page numbers, year of publication, and usually an abstract. When an article is submitted to MEDLINE for inclusion, subject specialists read each article and classify the article using standardized vocabulary terms called Medical Subject Headings (MeSH). This classification system allows for all articles addressing a particular subject to be indexed under the same MeSH term. Typically, 15 to 20 MeSH terms are assigned for each article. The MeSH vocabulary includes more than 19,000 terms. For example Figure 2–6 displays the MEDLINE subject headings for the following citation: van Rensburg CJ, Hartmann M, Thorpe A, Venter

MeSH Subject Headings
> Adult
> Aged
> Aged, 80 and over
> *Anti-Ulcer Agents / ad [Administration & Dosage]
> *Benzimidazoles / ad [Administration & Dosage]
> Female
> Gastrointestinal Hemorrhage / et [Etiology]
> *Gastrointestinal Hemorrhage / pc [Prevention & Control]
> Gastroscopy
> Human
> Hydrogen-Ion Concentration
> **Infusions**, Intravenous
> Male
> Middle Aged
> *Peptic Ulcer / co [Complications]
> Peptic Ulcer / th [Therapy]
> Pilot Projects
> Prospective Studies
> Recurrence
> *Sulfoxides / ad [Administration & Dosage]
> Support, Non-U.S. Gov't
> Treatment Outcome

Figure 2-6
MeSH subject headings for a specific MEDLINE citation.

L, Theron I, Luhmann R, Wurst W. Intragastric pH during continuous **infusion** with **panto-prazole** in patients with bleeding peptic ulcer. *Am J Gastroenterol.* 2003;98(12):2635–41.

Reading the MeSH terms tells us that this article is about a human (could be female or male, no children were included) being treated to prevent or treat peptic ulcer disease. From the MeSH terms we are able to deduce that this article describes a pilot prospective study in which subjects with gastrointestinal hemorrhage or peptic ulcer (both terms are emphasized with an asterisk, indicating that they are a primary focus of the article) received an antiulcer agent via intravenous infusion, and their hydrogen-ion concentration was measured. The "/ th" further classifies the MeSH term into the therapy category. For example "peptic ulcer / th" means that the article is about the therapy of peptic ulcer. When a MEDLINE search is performed, the system automatically tries to match the selected terms or elements to the MeSH terms that are assigned to the millions of articles included in the database. This process is referred to as mapping.

The basic steps involved in each search are as follows: (1) Identify key elements from a well-formulated question that can be used within the search strategy as MeSH terms or text words; (2) combine terms using Boolean operators ("AND," "OR," and "NOT"); (3) refine the search

---

User Tip

The MeSH vocabulary includes the terms below for designating the ages of persons. When an article is indexed, one or more of these headings may be assigned. In this example, the terms "adult," "middle aged," and "aged, 80 and over" were assigned to the article.

1. Infant (birth to 23 months)
2. Child (birth to 18 years)
3. Adolescence (13–18 years)
4. Adult (19 years and over)
5. Middle age (45–64 years)
6. Aged (65 years and over)
7. Aged, 80 and over (80 years and over)

using predefined limits (human subjects, publication type, search filters); and (4) improve the search strategy on the basis of retrieved citations.

Scenario

The intensive care unit (ICU) nurse calls you at the pharmacy: Dr. GI prescribed Protonix iv (pantoprazole—Wyeth-Ayerst Laboratories) for continuous infusion at 8 mg per hour, but a reference book available on the ICU says the drug should be given as bolus doses once or twice daily. The nurse asks if you can call and have the order changed.

As you investigate further (on the basis of your skills to better formulate a focused question), you find out that the patient is a 65-year-old man who presented with a bleeding peptic ulcer. The ICU physician consulted the gastroenterology service, and one of those physicians wrote the order for the continuous pantoprazole infusion.

Formulating the Question

Remember the generic question: In this Patient, is the Intervention better, worse, or equivalent to the Comparison to prevent or treat the Outcome?

In this 65-year-old man with an active bleeding peptic ulcer, can pantoprazole be administered as a continuous infusion instead of twice daily to suppress acid production?

Identifying the Search Terms

One of the most important steps in the literature search is to analyze the question and identify the terms that can be used as MeSH terms or text words in the search strategy (Figure 2–7). In general, key elements that are essential in a search strategy include (1) the patient condition or the disease (the limit option may be helpful) and (2) the intervention of interest. Even though components of the question such as the comparison and the outcomes are also important, these concepts are often not well indexed by MEDLINE.

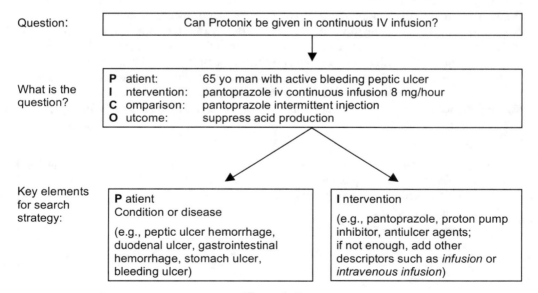

Figure 2-7

Basic steps in identifying key MeSH terms or text words. IV = Intravenous.

User Tip

To do a text-word search, enter the term followed by the extension ".tw.": for example, "panto-prazole.tw." or "(bleeding ulcer).tw." The extension tells the system to search for that word or phrase in the titles and abstracts of the citations. Using the $ symbol in Ovid and * in PubMed can truncate text-word searches. Truncation allows one to search for variations of words:

> interven$.tw. for "intervene" or "intervened" or "intervention"
> Child*.tw. for "child" or "children"

If age group is a key element of the question, use the limit option of the main search screen. A limit focuses the search on a certain aspect of information contained in a record such as age groups, publication year or type (e.g., review article, meta-analysis, language). Limits vary from database to database but this option, when available, makes the search easier.

It is always a good approach to identify multiple terms or synonyms that describe the condition or disease (e.g., peptic ulcer hemorrhage, bleeding ulcer, upper gastrointestinal hemorrhage) and terms describing the intervention (e.g., proton pump inhibitor or pantoprazole). To have the system automatically suggest synonyms, the user can type the term in the search box. Figure 2–8 illustrates how MEDLINE attempted to map "bleeding ulcer" to a list of known MeSH terms that may be synonyms before searching for it as a text word. The use of quotation marks or wildcard symbols will turn off this automatic mapping. For example, use of the phrase "breast cancer" will retrieve those records using that phrase, but the records indexed according to the MeSH term "breast neoplasms" will be omitted.

In general, both MeSH terms and text words should be used to develop a comprehensive search strategy. Text-word searching is better than MeSH for (1) proper names (Palmaz–Schatz stents) or (2) terms that are too new (new technology, drug in development) to be indexed or rare enough that they were likely used. Text-word searching is weak for terms that have a lot of synonyms because the search retrieves only citations containing the selected key word.

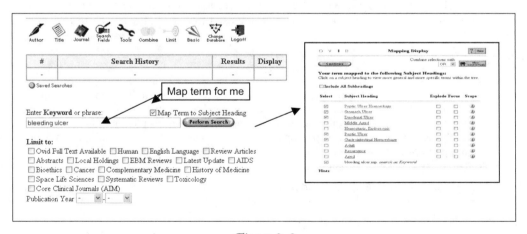

Figure 2-8

Mapping a term in MEDLINE. Selected keywords: peptic ulcer hemorrhage, stomach ulcer, duodenal ulcer, peptic ulcer, gastrointestinal hemorrhage, and bleeding ulcer as a text word. (Copyright Ovid Technologies and Wolters Kluwer Health, reproduced with permission.)

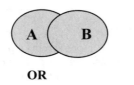
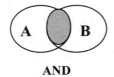
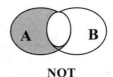

OR   **AND**   **NOT**

Figure 2–9
Boolean operators and their logic.

Combine Terms Using Boolean Logic

MEDLINE uses three Boolean operators: "AND," "OR," and "NOT." The "OR" Boolean operator will return all the articles that address A only, all articles that address B only, and all articles that address A and B. The "AND" Boolean operator will return only articles that contain both A and B. The "NOT" Boolean operator will return only articles that address A, and will eliminate articles that address B only and articles that address A and B (Figure 2–9).

Unlike the other two operators, the order of the sets joined by the operator "NOT" is important. In general, the resultant set will contain documents from the first set, but will exclude those documents that are also found in the second set.

Once the key terms for a search is identified (terms describing the condition or disease of interest including all possible synonyms), the Boolean operators "AND" and "OR" are used to combine the terms. In general the synonyms are combined by using "OR." For example, if articles addressing management of bleeding ulcers are of interest and the mapping tool in MEDLINE found synonyms, the terms can be combined with "OR" (Figure 2–10). The new search result contains all the articles in all the original sets but the duplicates are eliminated.

Use of the operator "AND" narrows the results retrieved from MEDLINE. The terms describing the condition are combined, and only the articles that address both the condition *and* the intervention of interest are excluded (Figure 2–11).

In the previous example, MEDLINE retrieved more than 2000 articles. This search is likely comprehensive but not very precise. To increase search specificity, one can add new terms (concepts) to the search strategy. In this case, the specific question relates to a delivery mode (continuous infusion compared with intermittent injection), so terms for these modes can be added to the search, and Boolean operators can be used to narrow the search to the specific articles of interest (Figure 2–12).

User Tip

Boolean operators can get tricky. According to PubMed/MEDLINE rules, when several Boolean operators are used in a search strategy, they are read from left to right. In the following statements, statement 1 returns all articles addressing peptic ulcer or bleeding ulcer and then combines the search with the term "pantoprazole," while statement 2 returns all articles either addressing pantoprazole and peptic ulcer or addressing bleeding ulcer. Search strategy 2 will result in a number of unwanted hits.

1. Peptic ulcer or bleeding ulcer and pantoprazole
2. Pantoprazole and peptic ulcer or bleeding ulcer

The following steps can resolve this problem:

➤ Remember the left-to-right rule.
➤ Group terms in parentheses.
➤ Or for each combination, create a command line and then combine them.

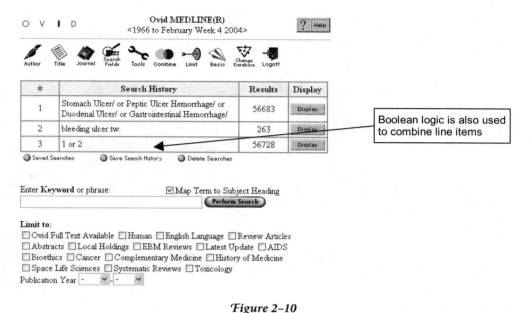

Figure 2-10
Use of Boolean operators to combine terms.
(Copyright Ovid Technologies and Wolters Kluwer Health, reproduced with permission.)

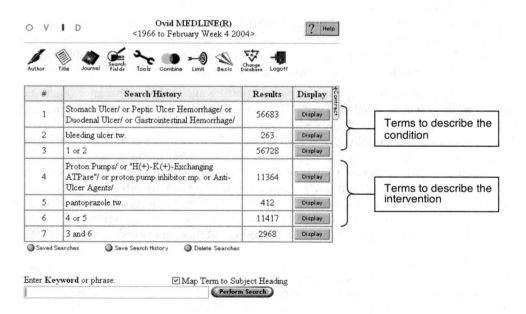

Figure 2-11
Use of Boolean term "AND" to narrow search results.
(Copyright Ovid Technologies and Wolters Kluwer Health, reproduced with permission.)

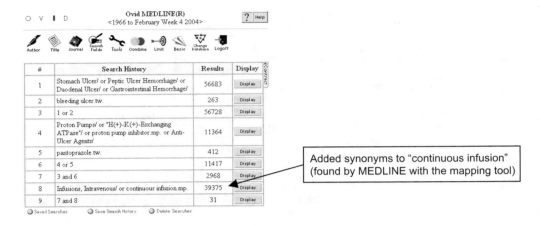

Figure 2–12
Use of additional terms to refine search.
(Copyright Ovid Technologies and Wolters Kluwer Health, reproduced with permission.)

Methods to Refine Searches

Use of Adjacency Operators
A commonly used operator is the adjacency operator. Terms or abbreviation used for adjacency include "NEAR," "ADJ," and "SAME":

> ➤ ADJ: Finds citations that contain the search terms right next to each other or within "n" words of each other.
> ➤ NEAR: Finds citations that contain the search terms right next to each other, but in any order. Depending on the database, the terms might also be in the same sentence.
> ➤ SAME: Finds citations that contain the search terms in the same paragraph, same field, or same sentence (depending on the database used).

The operator allows a more specific search by ensuring that the two terms are close to each other or within a specific number of words. For example, the search "patient* ADJ3 education" will find the words "patient(s)" and "education" within three words of each other in either direction. This approach would retrieve documents with phrases such as "pharmacy programs offering education for patients with hypertension," "patient education programs offered by pharmacists," "pharmacists involved in the education of hypertensive patients," and so forth.

"ADJ" is ideal for the search in which the researcher is not exactly sure of the phraseology that may have been used in the literature. Also, requiring two or more search terms to be near each other will usually retrieve documents in which the terms are closely related.

Some databases, including PubMed, do not allow use of these operators.

Use of Predefined Limits to Refine Search
Most databases offer a method of setting limits to restrict the number of citations retrieved in a search. For example, a search of Ovid for only randomized controlled trials done in humans, more specifically male, published in English between 1999 and 2004 would involve the limit fields highlighted in Figure 2–13. This figure displays all the limit fields that exist in the Ovid interface. Similar limits also exist for PubMed. Placing limits on the search strategy decreases the number of citations one needs to review and focuses the search on the most relevant articles.

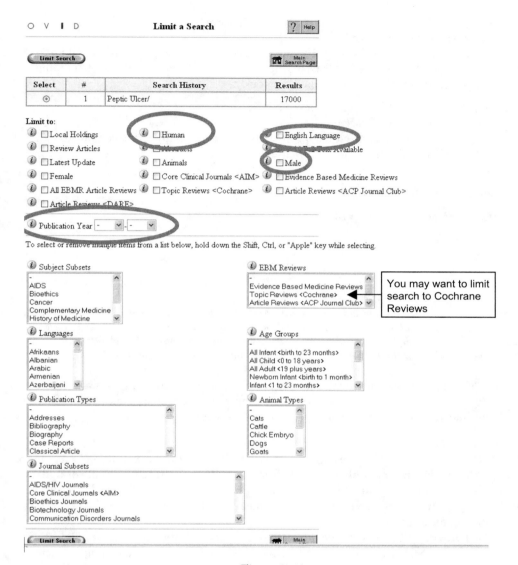

Figure 2-13
Use of Ovid interface to limit a search.
(Copyright Ovid Technologies and Wolters Kluwer Health, reproduced with permission.)

Use of Retrieved Citations to Improve Search Strategy
Reviewing the MeSH subject headings and reading the abstracts of the retrieved citations will provide additional synonyms that may help refine a search strategy. This technique is called "bootstrapping." Reviewing the references of articles to capture additional citations that may have been missed is called "pearling."

Troubleshooting Electronic Searches

Two primary problems with electronic searches are retrieval of irrelevant results or no results.

> *Problem 1.* Most of the citations retrieved are irrelevant.
> *Solution:* Focus the search.
> —Are the terms specific enough? Were terms combined (using synonyms and Boolean logic)? Explore MeSH terms to help define search terms. Use the bootstrapping and pearling techniques described previously.

> *Problem 2.* No citations were retrieved by the search.
> *Solution:* Broaden the search.
> —Was "AND" or "OR" used inappropriately? Were too many terms combined with "AND"? Was the "explode" feature used?

Additional Tips on Electronic Searches

Single Citation Matcher From PubMed

∽
Scenario
∽

You receive a call at the drug information center from one of the prominent researchers in the field of diabetes. Dr. D. is on a deadline to finish his National Institutes of Health submission and needs a reference he simply cannot find. He remembers that Dr. Lakka is one author and the article is about metabolic syndrome and mortality. He thinks it was published in 2002, but he just cannot remember in which journal.

The PubMed citation matcher (available on the side toolbar; Figure 2–14) allows the user to search for an incomplete or incorrect citation by simply filling out at least one of the following fields: journal, date, volume, issue, first page, author, or text in the title.

Saving a Search Strategy
All MEDLINE platforms allow searches to be saved. This tool can help clinicians keep up to date. For example, on a monthly or weekly basis a clinician can receive e-mails of updated MEDLINE search results and review what is new in a field of interest. For pharmacists conducting systematic reviews, saving the search strategy enables them to update their reviews as new data become available.

PubMed provides all users with the option to register in the National Center for Biotechnology Information (NCBI). At no charge, NCBI allows the user to store saved searches and create "auto e-mail alerts" every day, week, or month when there are new publications for the saved search (Figure 2–15).

Applying Filters to Optimize Searches
PubMed offers specialized searches using methodologic filters. These filters, based on work by Haynes and colleagues,[9] are validated search strategies designed to identify the best clinically relevant studies that answer questions about etiology, prognosis, diagnosis, or treatment of a disease. The user can select to emphasize the search on sensitivity to find the most citations on a topic, meaning that less relevant citations will be captured by this filter. Or the user may elect to emphasize the search on specificity to find only the most relevant citations. The terms used for the filters can be found at http://www.cebm.net/searching.asp. The filters are also offered by most other platforms for MEDLINE.

Step 1. Enter date, author's last name, and title words

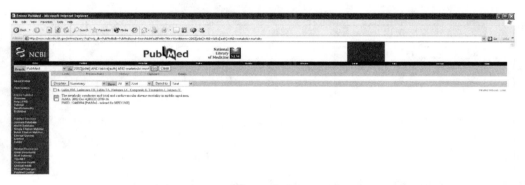

Step 2. Single citation manager found following article

Figure 2–14
Citation matcher feature of PubMed.

Finding Information on the World Wide Web

～
Scenario
～

Mrs. Jane, a well-known patient at your pharmacy, was just diagnosed with endometriosis. She says that her physician explained to her what the disease is, but she would like more information. Can you help her?

The World Wide Web (WWW) provides an endless supply of resources. Basing treatment decisions on or passing information from the WWW to patients may be risky though. All information published on the WWW is not accurate. There are three basic questions to ask while judging the accuracy and validity of a WWW resource:

➢ Who has provided the information (authors' credentials)? (Uniform resource locator [URL] extensions indicate the source of information in a broad sense: ".com" suggests a commercial entity, ".org" suggests a nonprofit organization, ".edu" suggests an academic institution, and ".gov" suggests a government department.)

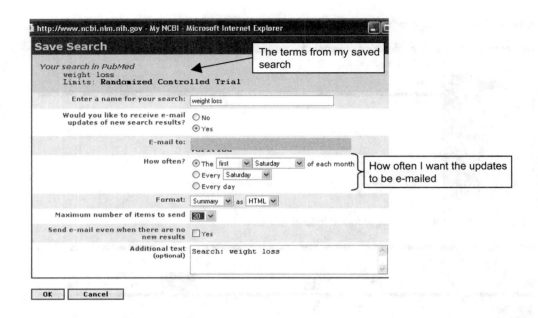

Figure 2-15
National Center for Biotechnology Information auto e-mail alert for saved search.

> When was it created/published/last updated (is it up-to-date)?
> Where is the information coming from (is the source of the information known)? A great tutorial for pharmacists on how to search the Internet is available at http://www. vts.rdn.ac.uk/tutorial/pharmacist/?sid=2361583&op=preview&manifestid=127&itemid= 12477.)

Three Types of Search Tools (Table 2–4)

Search Engines The search engines (e.g., Google, Lycos, Altavista) include no human intervention or quality control. These are programs that search the pages indexed. Therefore, using a search engine is not searching the entire WWW.

Metasearch Engines To facilitate the searches of multiple Internet sources, metasearch engines are useful. Metasearch tools launch a single query across a set of Web-based health sites. One query returns a merged and often ranked list of hits, allowing the user to search several databases at once. Table 2–5 describes the specifics of new metasearch engines available to search for Internet-based health information.

Subject Gateways Subject gateways are also called "subject guides," "subject directories," or "information gateways." They are directories of Web pages and documents, and Web sites on a given topic. The quality and size of the directories vary, but the best subject gateways assess the

Table 2-4 Internet Search Tools

Description	Strengths	Weakness	Examples
Search engines	Huge indexes of Web sites that often retrieve a lot of information.	The indexes are created by robots or spiders and are unevaluated. Reader must evaluate all information.	http://www.google.com http://www.search.yahoo.com http://www.ask.com (merged with teoma.com) http://www.lycos.com http://www.hotbot.com
Metasearch engines	Searches quickly and superficially several individual search engines at once.	They tend to return results from smaller and/or free search engines and miscellaneous free directories.	http://www.metacrawler.com http://www.ixquick.com http://www.surfwax.com http://www.northernlight.com http://www.copernic.com http://www.webcrawler.com http://www.vivisimo.com (searches Netscape, MSM, Lycos, looksmart, and more) http://www.dogpile.com (searches Google, Yahoo, Altavista, Teoma and Ask Jeeves, about.com, Looksmart, and more)
Subject directories/ gateways	High quality and most are evaluated. Of great value when doing academic research.	Collection is small.	http://www.rdn.ac.uk http://www.scout.wisc.edu/Archives http://www.britannica.com http://www.vlib.org http://www.lii.org http://infomine.ucr.edu http://www.academicinfo.net http://www.about.com/
The invisible Web	Collection of specialized databases that cannot be indexed by search engines. Is estimated to offer twice as many pages as the visible Web.	Can be hard to use.	http://www.internettutorials.net/deepweb.html (provides tutorial on accessing invisible Web) http://www.freepint.com http://www.eduref.org http://www.pubmed.org/query.fcgi http://www.doaj.org

quality of the resource before including them in the directory. The information obtained can be more reliable than that found with a search engine.

For this scenario, the term "endometriosis" was searched on Health On the Net (http://www.hon.ch). The search directed the user to the MEDLINEPlus Web site, which offered a patient-oriented tutorial to better understand endometriosis (to be viewed as either a slide show or printed material).

Table 2–5 Metasearch Engines for Web-Based Health Information

Resource Description	Special Features
Turning Research Into Practice (TRIP) (http://www.tripdatabase.com) Includes 58 sources, including sites for top 20 medical journals, EBM sites such as Bandolier, critically appraised bank, Cochrane Database of Systematic Review, A Journal Club on the Web, EBM series, guidelines, and systematic review sites such as SIGN, DARE, NICE, and the National Guideline Clearinghouse.	Monthly updates; uses keywords in the title only; subscription required. Results displayed by categories as evidence-based, peer-reviewed journals, guidelines, or other.
SUMSearch (http://SUMSearch.uthscsa.edu) Contains three Internet sites: The National Library of Medicine, DARE, and the National Guideline Clearinghouse.	Uses metasearch and contingency search techniques to requery the sites if the first search resulted in too many or too few hits.
Search.com (http://www.search.com) Includes 22 Internet sites containing health and medical information. Examples are American College of Physician Online, Centers for Disease Control and Prevention, New England Journal of Medicine, Agency for Healthcare Research and Quality, JAMA, PubMed, Merck, Mayo Clinic, Food and Drug Administration, World Health Organization, WebMD, and MeSH. It selects the best resources among several full-text books and biomedical databases for the question, formats the question for each resource, and makes additional searches on the basis of results. Dr. Robert Badgett developed this resource at the University of Texas Health Science Center at San Antonio.	Allows customization in choosing search engines and how to display results.
Federated Query Server (http://queryserver.com) Includes 12 sites containing health and medical information: American Health Consultants, American Heart Association, Centers for Disease Control and Prevention, Department of Health and Human Services, Food and Drug Administration, Johns Hopkins Infectious Diseases, Leukemia and Lymphoma Society, MEDLINE, Medscape Clinical Content, Medscape News, National Institutes of Health, and National Library of Medicine.	Results sorted according to content and/or source.
HON (Health On the Net) (http://www.hon.ch) HON developed Medhunt, a specialized search engine dedicated to medical Web pages (searches the full text of more than 60,000 documents). HON also offers HON Select to search medical information using the MeSH index. It searches several high-quality databases, including MEDLINE, Clinitrials.gov, news Web sites, and media gallery for medical images.	Results sorted by MEDLINE article, Web resources, medical image, medical news, medical conference, and clinical trials.

EBM = Evidence-based medicine; SIGN = Scottish Intercollegiate Guidelines Network; DARE = Database of Abstracts of Reviews or Effectiveness; NICE = National Institute for Health and Clinical Excellence.

Source: Chiquette E, Posey LM. Evidence-based medicine. In: *Pharmacotherapy: A Pathophysiologic Approach.* DiPiro JT, Talbert RL, Yee GC, et al. New York: McGraw-Hill; 2005:31. Adapted with permission of The McGraw-Hill Companies. Copyright 2005.

The Bottom Line

Reformulate the Question

➤ Remember PICO (Patient, Intervention, Comparison, and Outcome).

MEDLINE Tips

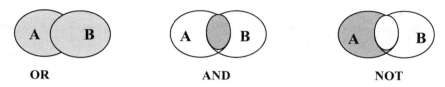

Boolean operators and their logic.

➤ If included, "AND," "OR," and "NOT" must be in uppercase.
➤ To truncate text-word searches, use $ in Ovid/MEDLINE and * in PubMed.
➤ Use "wom#n" to retrieve the words "woman" and "women" (# may be used for *one* character only).
➤ Use "colo?r" to retrieve the words "color" and "colour" (? may be used for one character or none).
➤ For an author search, enter last name, followed by a space and the first initial.
➤ Field labels include "TI" for title, "AU" for author, "AB" for abstract, and "TX" for full-text fields (includes title, abstract, subject headings).
➤ PreMEDLINE citations can be searched by using only text words.
➤ The Single Citation Matcher requires only a few elements of a citation to retrieve a complete PubMed citation:
  —Click on "Single Citation Matcher."
  —Enter the journal title, year, volume, issue, first page, or author's name. (Only one of these items has to be included.)

Additional Reading

McKibbon KA, Richardson WS, Walker DC. Finding answers to well built clinical questions. *Evidence Based Med.* 1999;6:164–7.

Hunt DL, Jaeschke R, McKibbon KA. Using electronic health information resources in evidence-based practice. The Evidence-Based Medicine Working Group. *JAMA.* 2000;283:1875–9.

Greenhalgh T. How to read a paper: the Medline database. *BMJ.* 1997;315:180–3.

References

1. Sackett DL, Richardson WS, Rosenberg WMC, Haynes RB, eds. *Evidence-Based Medicine: How to Practice and Teach EBM.* New York: Churchill Livingstone; 1997:7–9.

2. Richardson WS, Wilson MC, Nishikawa J, Hayward RSA. The well-built clinical question: a key to evidence-based decisions. *ACP J Club.* 1997;123:A12–3.

3. Bucher HC, Guyatt GH, Cook DJ, et al. Users' guides to the medical literature, XIX. Applying clinical trial results. A. How to use an article measuring the effect of an intervention on surrogate end points. Evidence-Based Medicine Working Group. *JAMA* 1999;282:771–8.

4. Ramsey PG, Carline JD, Inui TS, et al. Change over time in the knowledge base of practicing internists. *JAMA.* 1991;266:1103–7.

5. Mulrow CD. The medical review article: state of the science. *Ann Intern Med.* 1987;106:485–8.

6. Mulrow CD. Rationale for systematic reviews. *BMJ.* 1994;309;597–9.

7. Oxman A, Guyatt GH. The science of reviewing research. *Ann NY Acad Sci.* 1993;703:125–34.

8. Ebbert JO, Dupras DM, Erwin PJ. Searching the medical literature using PubMed: a tutorial. *Mayo Clin Proc.* 2003;78:87–91.

9. Haynes RB, Wilczynski N, McKibbon KA, et al. Developing optimal search strategies for detecting clinically sound studies in MEDLINE. *J Am Med Inform Assoc.* 1994;1:447–58.

APPENDIX 2–A
APPLY YOUR SEARCHING SKILLS

Web Tutorials

- ➤ Question formulation tutorial: http://www.cebm.utoronto.ca/practise
- ➤ PubMed tutorial: http://www.nlm.nih.gov/bsd/pubmed_tutorial/m1001.html
- ➤ Internet tutorial for pharmacists: http://itp.pharmacy.dal.ca/.
- ➤ ADEPT (Applying Diagnosis, Etiology, Prognosis & Therapy methodologic filters to retrieving the evidence). This is a Web tutorial developed by Andrew Booth, director of information at South Thames Regional Library, University of Sheffield. Review the material and complete the therapy exercise available at: http://www.shef.ac.uk/scharr/ir/adept/therapy/learn.htm.

Exercises

Scenario 1

You receive a call from a mother who wishes to mix metaproterenol sulfate (Alupent—Boehringer Ingelheim Pharmaceuticals, Inc.) in her infant's milk/formula.

Reframe the question

P:

I:

C:

O:

Suggestion: Does infant milk/formula interact with the absorption of metaproterenol sulfate? (P: infant; I: Alupent; C: not applicable; O: absorption of metaproterenol sulfate)

Question type

Background question ☐   *or*   Foreground question ☐

Search the following tools

Tool	Findings
Package insert	
Micromedex Healthcare Series (http://www.micromedex.com/products/hcs)	
Pediatric Dosage Handbook	
Other: name a source	

Answer

Neither food nor milk interacts with metaproterenol (information found in Micromedex Healthcare Series).

Scenario 2

One of your customers who has a 1-year-old infant wants to know at what age she can give the child ibuprofen suspension.

Reframe the question

P:

I:

C:

O:

Suggestion: Is it safe to give ibuprofen suspension to a 1-year-old infant? (P: 1-year-old infant; I: ibuprofen suspension; C: not applicable; O: toxicity)

Question type

Background question □   *or*   Foreground question □

Search the following tools

Tool	Findings
Package insert	
Pediatric Dosage Handbook	
Rxlist.com (http://www.rxlist.com)	

Answer

Yes, dosage guidelines are given for 6-month-old and older infants.

Scenario 3

You receive a call from an emergency room nurse who needs help identifying a white and blue tablet. You ask about the shape of the tablet and if there is any visible writing or markings. The nurse states that the tablet is a pale blue color, round, and has "MD" on one side and "530" on the other.

Reframe the question

P:

I:

C:

O:

Suggestion: What is the active ingredient and strength of the pale blue, round tablet with the codes "MD" and "530"?

(P: not applicable; I: pale blue, round tablet with codes "MD" and "530"; C: none; O: active ingredient)

Question type:

Background question   ☐   *or*   Foreground question   ☐

Search the following tools

Tool	Findings
Micromedex Healthcare Series (http://www.micromedex.com/products/hcs)	
Physicians' Desk Reference	
Internet (terms: "md530" versus "blue md530 tablet")	
Drugs.com (http://drugs.com; pill identification wizard)	

Answer

Methylphenidate hydrochloride 10 mg (various manufacturers)

Scenario 4

You receive a call from an internist in clinic. He describes a 45-year-old woman with signs and symptoms of irritable bowel syndrome (IBS) and asks what the best therapy is. He heard about tegaserod (Zelnorm—Novartis Pharmaceuticals Corp.), but asks if it is any better than a diet high in fiber or the antispasmodic agents.

Reframe the question

P:

I:

C:

O:

Suggestion: In patients with IBS, what are the most effective therapies? (P: 45-year-old- woman with IBS; I: tegaserod or antispasmodic agents or bulking agents; C: placebo or head to head; O: improvement in symptoms)

Question type

Background question ☐   *or*   Foreground question ☐

Search the following tools

Tool	Findings
ACP Journal Club	
PubMed (http://www.pubmed.org)	
UpToDate (http://www.uptodate.com)	

Answer

The results of a systematic review report that, in patients with IBS, tegaserod improves IBS symptoms in patients with constipation, and alosetron (Lotronex—GlaxoSmithKline) improves IBS symptoms in those with diarrhea.

Scenario 5

A nurse at a local nursing home calls to inquire about the compatibility of scopolamine and morphine. You investigate further and find that a 70-year-old man with terminal cancer is receiving morphine, scopolamine, lorazepam, and Robinul (glycopyrrolate—various manufacturers) via a subcutaneous butterfly device. Can morphine and scopolamine be mixed?

Reframe the question

P:
I:
C:
O:

Suggestion: What is the compatibility of morphine and scopolamine?

(P: 70-year-old man with a subcutaneous butterfly device; I: Can morphine and scopolamine be mixed, or should they be given separately? C: not applicable; O: to prevent interference with the pharmacokinetic and/or pharmacodynamic effect of either agent)

Question type:
Background question ☐   *or*   Foreground question ☐

Search the following tools

Tool	Findings
Trissel's *Handbook on Injectable Drugs*	
Handbook of Parenteral Drug Administration (http://members.ozemail.com.au/~jamesbc)	
King Guide to Parenteral Admixtures	
Micromedex Healthcare Series (http://www.micromedex.com/products/hcs)	

Answer
The products are physically compatible for at least 15 to 30 minutes.

Scenario 6

A doctor calls and wants to know the best treatment for *Bulkholderia cepacia*? After asking a few more questions you find out that an 18-year-old adolescent boy with cystic fibrosis was admitted to the hospital with pneumonia. The cultures returned positive for *B. cepacia*. What is the treatment?

Reframe the question

P:

I:

C:

O:

P: 18-year-old with cystic fibrosis with community-acquired pneumonia; positive for *B. cepacia;* I: What is the intervention? C: not applicable; O: eradicate *B. cepacia.*

Question type:
Background question   ☐   *or*   Foreground question   ☐

Search the following tools

Tool	Findings
The Sanford Guide to Antimicrobial Therapy	
Micromedex Healthcare Series (http://www.micromedex.com/products/hcs)	

Answer
Trimethoprim/sulfamethoxazole (various manufacturers) 5 mg/kg every 6 hours (first choice)
Meropenem (Merrem—Astra Pharma Pharmaceuticals, LP) 2 grams every 8 hours (second choice)

Scenario 7

A patient comes to the emergency department with a vial of Nobligan, which she bought in Mexico. She would like to be prescribed with the same medication. According to the patient it was relieving her pain well.

Reframe the question

P:

I:

C:

O:

Suggestion: What is the active ingredient in Nobligan?

(P: not applicable; I: Nobligan; C: not applicable; O: active ingredient)

Question type

Background question   □   *or*   Foreground question   □

Search the following tools

Tool	Findings
P.R. Vademecum ON-LINE http://www.prvademecum.com	
PJ Online http://www.pharmj.com/noticeboard/info/pip/ foreignmedicines.html	
Micromedex Healthcare Series (http://www.micromedex.com/products/hcs)	

Answer

Tramadol

Scenario 8

A physician wants to prescribe diclofenac (various manufacturers) and lithium (various manufacturers). He wants to know if these medications interact.

Reframe the question

P:

I:

C:

O:

Suggestion: Is diclofenac safer than other nonsteroidal anti-inflammatory drugs (NSAIDs) when combined with lithium?

(P: a patient already taking lithium; I: Is diclofenac a better choice? C: compared with other NSAIDs such as ibuprofen; O: to prevent drug interaction)

Search the following tools

Tool	Findings
Medscape (http://www.medscape.com/druginfo; registration is free)	
Micromedex Healthcare Series (http://www.micromedex.com/products/hcs)	
King Guide to Parenteral Admixtures	

Answer

Similar to other NSAIDs, diclofenac may increase lithium concentrations by 26%. If diclofenac is added, lithium concentrations should be monitored closely.

APPENDIX 2–B

RESOURCES FOR LOCATING EVIDENCE-BASED MEDICAL INFORMATION

Tutorials and other formats present search strategies for systematic reviews and meta-analyses. The major resources are listed here.

- ➤ The BMJ Publishing Group offers a very readable and practical series on MEDLINE searches in print and on the Internet. The series was originally published in the *British Medical Journal* and edited by Trisha Greenhalgh. A book is also now available.
  —The Medline database. *BMJ*. 1997;315:180–3.
  —http://www.bmj.com/cgi/content/full/315/7101/180.

- ➤ The Centre for Reviews and Dissemination also offers search strategies to identify systematic reviews and meta-analyses in MEDLINE databases at the following Web site:
  —http://www.york.ac.uk/inst/crd/search.htm.

- ➤ The Delfini Group, Inc. are consultants offering training in evidence-based medicine who have developed an excellent Web site with tools for every step of the search. The following URL leads to a Word document/handout that summarizes the key points of a well-conducted search of the medical literature including primary and secondary sources:
  —http://www.delfini.org/Delfini_Tool_Searching.doc.

- ➤ A superb hands-on Ovid tutorial, created by Connie Schardt, Education Coordinator for the Medical Center Library at Duke University, is available at:
  —http://www.mclibrary.duke.edu/training/ovid/home.

- ➤ The University of Sidney Library created a tutorial to search EMBASE, International Pharmaceutical Abstracts, and Medline. Also, the site offers handouts for how to search the Internet for pharmacy information and general information about evidence-based medicine, all for free:
  —http://www.library.usyd.edu.au/subjects/pharmacy/tutorials/embase/index.html.

- ➤ This tutorial from the University of North Carolina at Chapel Hill is designed to teach how to best select and search key resources (UpToDate, Cochrane Database of Systematic Reviews, *ACP Journal Club*, and PubMed) in locating evidence-based information. Each example includes screen captures of the respective database, making the learning experience more concrete:
  —http://www.hsl.unc.edu/Services/Tutorials/EBM_searching/pages/Welcome.htm.

- ➤ Lamar Soutter Library at the University of Massachusetts Medical School has developed a comprehensive online tutorial for evidence-based medicine, which also includes PowerPoint presentations on EBM:
  —http://library.umassmed.edu/EBM.

- ➤ A Cochrane Library tour developed by the National Electronic Library for Health. The recorded presentation by Kate Light provides comments at the same time the slides and screen captures of the Cochrane Library are viewed:
  —http://www.nelh.nhs.uk/tour/cochrane/cochrane1.asp?script=cochrane&slide=0.

MATCHING THE QUESTION WITH THE BEST AVAILABLE EVIDENCE

Elaine Chiquette and L. Michael Posey

*I*N CHAPTER 2, THE PROCESS OF IDENTIFYING RELEVANT STUDIES, GUIDELINES, AND STATE-MENTS was presented. But what happens when the evidence provided by these publications does not point toward the same or even similar treatments? Once the evidence has been identified, the next task—which is the subject of this chapter—is to evaluate the evidence and to determine whether the evidence offered by some studies should be valued more than that from other trials.

Clinical studies use a variety of methodologic approaches to test various therapeutic modalities, determine what behaviors and chemicals might be associated with disease, and assess whether adverse outcomes are linked to medications or demographic or clinical characteristics. Some of these approaches are considered stronger than others, and the strength of the evidence is important in determining the best course of action for individual patients.

Rappelling the Mountain of Evidence

Randomization was developed as a research method by R. A. Fisher in 1923 to compare the effect of fertilizers on potato fields. In 1948, the *British Medical Journal* published what is considered the earliest modern randomized controlled trial (RCT) in medicine, which evaluated the effect of streptomycin for tuberculosis. Randomized controlled trials remain the gold standard for evaluating efficacy and safety of treatments. Occasionally, the evidence that a treatment is effective is apparent without needing to conduct an RCT. For example, a randomized trial is not necessary to show that transfusing blood into someone with severe hemorrhage is valuable or that wearing a parachute before jumping from a plane will increase survival and reduce lower extremities injuries.[1] Unfortunately, such clearly effective treatments are uncommon.

More commonly, RCTs have helped to confirm the value of many therapeutic options today and disproved or clarified the usefulness of others. For example, in 1970 observational studies had indicated a possible association between the occurrence of premature ventricular contractions (PVCs) in patients after myocardial infarction (MI) and sudden death. As a result, the eighth edition of *Harrison's Principles of Internal Medicine* recommended the use of antiarrhythmic agents to eradicate post-MI PVCs and thereby minimize the risk of sudden death.

However, antiarrhythmic therapy was tested later in patients with frequent PVCs; the results showed that class I antiarrhythmic agents increased rather than decreased the risk of sudden death.[2,3] Today guidelines discourage the use of antiarrhythmic agents to suppress PVCs in post-MI patients.[4]

More recently, the 1996 guidelines for the management of patients with acute MI concluded that observational studies "indicate that estrogen therapy does reduce mortality in women with moderate and severe coronary disease."[5] Subsequently, RCTs found no reduction in overall risk for nonfatal MI or coronary death with estrogen therapy.[6-8] Rather, significantly more coronary events occurred during the first year of the trial among women receiving estrogen therapy compared with women taking placebo. These results prompted revision of the guidelines as follows: "On the basis of the findings postmenopausal women should not receive combination estrogen and progestin therapy for primary or secondary prevention of CHD. It is recommended that the use of hormone therapy be discontinued in women who have myocardial infarction."[4]

In both of these examples, conventional wisdom was wrong. Results from observational studies proved incorrect. Only through careful assessment using RCT methodology was the true estimate of the efficacy and safety of the therapeutic options discovered.

RCTs, however, cannot answer all clinical questions, such as situations in which RCTs may not be appropriate or ethical. For instance, a trial in which consenting pregnant women are randomized to receive either tetracycline or a placebo to assess teratogenicity is unethical. Also, because RCTs are more expensive and complicated to conduct than other types of studies, only rarely is one available to answer a very specific question. Therefore, clinicians must rely on other types of study designs to answer some of their clinical questions. The key is to pick the best available evidence that exists to answer a question, as shown in Table 3–1.

Climbing the Evidence Ladder

All evidence is not created equal (see Appendix 3–A for a detailed description of major clinical trial designs). Table 3–2 summarizes the advantages and disadvantages of different trial designs.

Table 3–1 Different Types of Questions Require Different Types of Evidence

Types/Examples of Questions	Types of Studies Likely to Yield Evidence
Therapy: Can rosuvastatin (Crestor—AstraZeneca Pharmaceuticals) prevent cardiovascular events in participants with dyslipidemia?	≻ Systematic review of RCTs ≻ RCT
Harm: Does diltiazem increase the risk of cancer?	≻ Systematic review of RCTs* ≻ RCT ≻ Cohort ≻ Case–control ≻ Systematic review of case reports
Compatibility: Can you mix insulin with TPN?	≻ In vitro studies
Drug interaction: Do statins interact with warfarin?	≻ Systematic review of case reports/case series ≻ Case reports/case series

RCT = Randomized controlled trial; TPN = total parenteral nutrition.

* Pooled analysis of RCTs can be useful, but frequently harmful effects are rare and not detected in short-term RCTs.

Table 3–2   Advantages and Disadvantages of Different Trial Designs

Trial Design	Advantages	Disadvantages
Randomized controlled trial 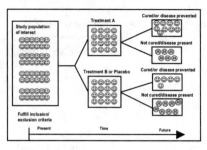	➢ Unbiased distribution of known and unknown confounders ➢ Blinding more likely ➢ Causability can be established	➢ Expensive: time and money ➢ Ethically problematic at times
Cohort study 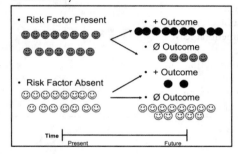	➢ Ethically safe ➢ Retrospective ➢ Can establish timing and directionality of events ➢ Eligibility criteria and outcome assessments can be standardized ➢ Administratively easier and cheaper than RCT	➢ Controls may be difficult to identify and match ➢ Exposure may be linked to a hidden confounder ➢ Blinding is difficult to impossible ➢ For rare diseases, large sample sizes or long follow-up is necessary ➢ Unable to randomize; therefore, distribution of unknown confounders may be unequal
Case–control studies 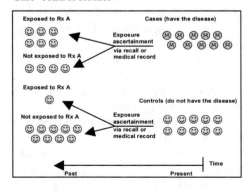	➢ Quick and cheap ➢ Most commonly retrospective ➢ Only feasible method for very rare disorders or those with long lag between exposure and outcome ➢ Fewer subjects needed than for cross-sectional studies ➢ Subjects should be matched	➢ Reliance on recall or records to determine exposure status ➢ Selection of control groups is difficult ➢ Establish association, not causality ➢ At risk for recall and selection bias ➢ Retrospective

Table 3–2 (continued)   Advantages and Disadvantages of Different Trial Designs

Trial Design	Advantages	Disadvantages
Cross-sectional study	➤ Cheap and simple ➤ Ethically safe ➤ Snapshot view	➤ Establish association, not causality ➤ At risk for recall bias ➤ Confounders may be unequally distributed
Crossover design	➤ All subjects serve as own controls and error variance is reduced, thus reducing sample size needed ➤ All subjects receive treatment (at least some of the time) ➤ Randomization can be used ➤ Blinding can be maintained	➤ Washout period lengthy or unknown ➤ Cannot be used for treatments with curative potential

The Evidence Ladder

Much of the debate about the evidence ladder concerns the studies placed at the top (Figure 3–1). Which is best: a meta-analysis or a mega trial? Mega trials are large-scale, randomized, controlled clinical trials recruiting thousands of patients from large numbers of trial sites with the aim of providing reliable evidence on clinical outcomes of treatment. Meta-analyses are usually conducted in areas for which a number of relatively small RCTs have produced conflicting conclusions. Different conclusions occur commonly as a result of studies having different inclusion and exclusion criteria, resulting in different populations of patients being studied.

In such a situation, authors of a meta-analysis seek to find clarity among seemingly divergent data. The meta-analysis may point clearly in one direction when the data from all pertinent RCTs are combined. Later, however, a mega trial is sometimes conducted to further elucidate the role of a treatment; further discrepancies can then be uncovered (Figure 3–2).[9,10]

One example of such divergence in the literature involves the use of magnesium in coronary care units. In 1991, a meta-analysis concluded that magnesium was effective in reducing death in patients with MI and that its use should be adopted as a standard practice.[11] The meta-analysis included 1300 patients and found a 55% risk reduction in death. But a few years later, a randomized clinical trial involving more than 50,000 patients found no benefit, and magnesium infusions ceased to have any role in coronary care units.[12]

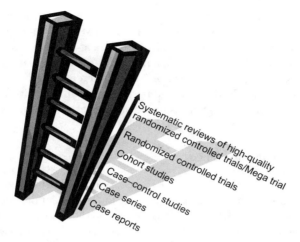

Figure 3-1

The evidence ladder. The weakest evidence for a question of efficacy and/or safety comes from case reports. Systematic reviews of high-quality randomized controlled trials and mega trials represent the evidence with the best design to answer a question about efficacy and/or safety of a given intervention. Several evidence-based medicine gurus would argue that systematic reviews of high-quality randomized controlled trials are the best evidence above mega trials. (Hierarchy is based on the levels of evidence presented by the Centre for Evidence-Based Medicine at http://www.cebm.net/levels_of_evidence.asp#levels.)

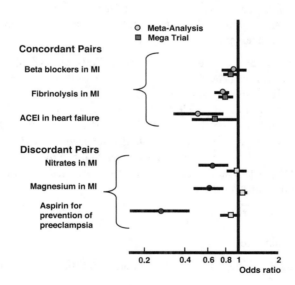

Figure 3-2

Meta-analysis versus mega trial. Examples of three interventions in which the mega trial confirmed the meta-analysis (*upper graph*) or refuted the results of the previous meta-analysis (*bottom graph*). The results are displayed as odds ratio (*circle* for meta-analysis; *square* for mega trial) and 95% CIs. (Adapted from Egger M, Davey Smith G, Schneider M, Minder C. Bias in meta-analysis detected by a simple, graphical test. *BMJ.* 1997;3;315(7109):629–34, Copyright (1997), with permission from BMJ Publishing Group.)

Several authors have attempted to explain the discrepancies between meta-analyses and subsequent mega trials. Two reviews[13,14] reported that most (80%) meta-analyses agreed with the results from their respective larger trials. However, meta-analyses may disagree with mega trials because meta-analyses include RCTs that involve different populations and different subgroups representing various patients' characteristics. Different subgroups may respond to the same therapy differently. In addition, individual trials use different inclusion and exclusion criteria. Furthermore, even two mega trials may disagree because of intrinsic variability.

Selecting the Best Available Evidence

To determine whether the identified evidence (a case report, cohort study, case–control analysis, or RCT) will help answer the clinical problem, one must consider the quality of the information. Poorly conducted trials and investigations that are on the low rungs of the evidence ladder may yield misleading results. In other words, one should not believe everything in the abstract of a published article. The following terms often are used to describe the quality of a trial:

> ➤ *External validity* refers to relevance, applicability, and generalizability: How likely is it that the results will occur in my patients, my hospital, my pharmacy? The external validity can be assessed usually by reviewing the inclusion/exclusion criteria of a trial.
> ➤ *Internal validity* addresses whether the conduct of the trial was conducted in such a way as to prevent as much error as possible, and therefore provide results that are accurate and the closest to the truth: How likely is it that the observed results were produced by the drug being studied?
> ➤ *Precision* and *validity* should not be confused. *Precision* is a measure of the likelihood of random errors. It is reflected in the confidence intervals around the estimates of each outcome measurement.

Critical appraisal methods must be used to assess validity of available studies. Worksheets for various types of studies are provided in Appendix 3–B of this chapter; they summarize the key considerations as discussed in detail in the following sections.

Appraisal is a technique to easily exclude research studies that are too poorly designed to influence one's practice. It is a structured checklist addressing the validity, reliability, and applicability of the study to an information need. This technique provides a tool to systematically evaluate the scientific literature, filter the studies that are methodologically sound, and help in deciding whether the results will influence one's practice. In other words, the critical appraisal techniques help answer three questions:

1. Are the results likely to be true?
2. What are the results?
3. Will it change what I do?

The first two questions are discussed in this chapter, and the third question is addressed in Chapter 5.

Scenario

During rounds, the cardiology resident asks you about the use of tegaserod (Zelnorm—Novartis Pharmaceuticals Corp.) for his patient. He read in the product labeling that the drug is indicated only for women, but he wants to know if it will work for treating irritable bowel syndrome in men. After questioning the resident further you formulate this question: Is tegaserod superior to placebo for reducing symptoms of bloating, abdominal pain, and constipation in a 57-year-old man with coronary artery disease and irritable bowel syndrome with predominant constipation symptoms? After rounds, you stop at a terminal with access to PubMed and do a quick search on tegaserod applying the limits "randomized controlled trial" and "male gender." You find 15 titles.

The first step in resolving the resident's query is to apply two screening questions:

1. Does each available study clearly define the question, and does it match the information needs? Simply reading the title can help eliminate half of the PubMed hits. Titles such as "the effects of tegaserod (HTF 919) on oesophageal acid exposure in gastro-oesophageal reflux disease" can be eliminated even before reading further.
2. Does the design of each available study match the information needs? The question being researched involves therapy. Therefore, the gold standard of evidence for therapy is a systematic review of RCTs. However, tegaserod is such a new medication that no systematic reviews yet exist. The next best trial design to answer this question is an RCT. PubMed lists more than five RCTs, which should provide plenty of evidence. Thus, further searches for other trial designs are unnecessary.

Once both questions have been answered affirmatively, the relevant articles can be pulled to appraise further the quality of the trial. The following section presents a series of questions pertinent to different trial designs that help assess the quality (internal validity) of various types of studies.

Assessing Validity of Randomized Controlled Trials[15]

The conduct of the trial should minimize systematic bias and random error as much as possible to ensure validity. The comparison of one treatment with another requires that the patients being compared are similar in all possible prognostically important ways except for the treatments under comparison. Four sources of bias are possible in therapy trials (Figure 3–3): selection bias, performance bias, attrition bias, and detection bias. Bias can result in an overestimation or underestimation of the effectiveness of a drug therapy and mislead the reader.

Was Subject Allocation Randomized?

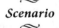

Scenario

In an attempt to review the impact of exercise on weight loss, you pulled an RCT from a 1994 issue of Medicine & Science in Sports & Exercise. The Methods section reads:

One hundred and thirty-eight sedentary nonsmoking Caucasian men older than 45 years who were between 120% and 160% of recommended body weight initially volunteered for participation in this investigation of the effects of weight loss and exercise training. Participants provided written informed consent. After the initial screening, participants had their body composition and maximal oxygen consumption measured. Participants were randomly assigned to one of three groups; however, individuals who refused their assignment were allowed to choose their intervention...

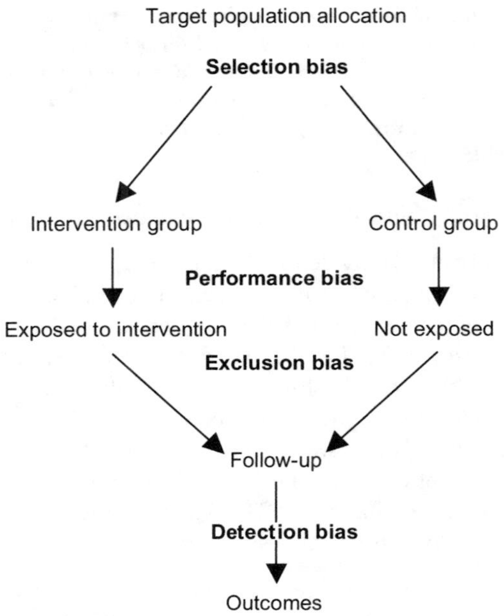

Figure 3-3

Most common sources of bias in trials addressing the efficacy and safety of drug therapy.

To minimize selection bias, researchers should ensure that all participants have an equal chance to be allocated to the treatment or control group. Randomization (i.e, researchers randomly assigned patients to the experimental treatment or control groups) is considered the best method to ensure that the known and unknown risk factors are equally distributed between the treatment and control groups. Random allocation means that each participant has the same chance of receiving each of the possible groups under investigation. If important risk factors known to affect prognosis (such as disease severity or presence of comorbidities) are unevenly distributed between groups, then selection bias could falsely estimate the benefit of the intervention. In the example above, randomization is sabotaged by the participants selecting their own assignments.

Tools to Minimize Selection Bias

Randomization   If two groups (an experimental treatment group and a control group) are involved, to randomize is to use a technique such as coin tossing that gives a 50–50 chance for the individual to be assigned to the experimental treatment group or to the control group. For example, subject A fulfills all inclusion and exclusion criteria, and has consented to participate in the trial. It is determined a priori that the subject be assigned to the experimental group if the result is "heads" or to the control group if the result is "tails." In practice, randomization is performed by using computer-generated randomization lists. This method is best to balance the groups for confounding factors.

Concealed Allocation   The subject's assignment (control or treatment group) should be concealed from the individual enrolling/recruiting the participants into the trial. Recruiters who assess eligibility criteria and are aware of the next random allocation may consciously or unconsciously select the healthiest patient to be enrolled in the control group or vice versa. For example,

> *User Tip*
>
> Confounding is the distortion of the effect of one risk factor by the presence of another. Confounding occurs when another risk factor for a disease is also associated with the risk factor being studied but acts separately. Examples of confounders may be age, gender, socioeconomic status, and so forth. Confounding bias is systematic error attributable to the failure to account for the effect of one or more variables that are related to both the causal factor being studied and the outcome, and are not distributed the same between the groups being studied.
>
> These factors may also be minimized by some form of stratification or adjustment procedure in the analysis. For example, if smoking is believed to be a confounding factor, the results can be examined separately in smokers and nonsmokers (stratification), or the results can be adjusted by calculations that consider different smoking habits (standardization).

the recruiter's preconceived idea is that the experimental drug will be good for patients with class I or class II heart failure, but may be too risky for those in class III (more advanced disease). Suppose the recruiter is enrolling a subject with class III heart failure, but learns that the subject would be assigned to treatment (according to the next random allocation). Consciously or unconsciously, the recruiter may influence the subject to refuse consent. Studies have shown that if randomization is not concealed, it tends to lead to patients with more favorable prognosis being given the experimental treatment, exaggerating the apparent benefits of therapy and possibly resulting in a conclusion that the treatment is efficacious when it is not.[16,17]

A randomization method is judged adequate if it allows each patient to have the same chance of receiving each treatment and prevents the investigators (or participants such as those in the scenario) from being able to predict which treatment allocation will be assigned next. Therefore, methods of allocation using date of birth, date of admission, hospital numbers, day or week, or open lists of random numbers are inadequate. For example, assigning to control groups all participants with an odd hospital number and to treatment groups all participants with an even hospital number would allow the investigator to know which group the participants will be assigned to. Examples of bias-free random allocations include centralized randomization (e.g., a central office unaware of subject characteristics allocates group assignments), pharmacy-controlled randomization (assuming the pharmacist is not recruiting the participants), prenumbered or coded identical containers that are administered serially to participants, or opaque envelopes (i.e., a recruiter/investigator cannot see through the envelope and read the allocation) that are sequentially numbered and sealed.

Successful Randomization   The ultimate test to determine the impact of possible selection bias is to review baseline characteristics for each group and assess whether significant differences exist between groups. Baseline characteristics that clearly show significant uneven distribution of important prognostic determinants imply that the randomization technique failed. Several reasons may have caused the randomization technique to result in an uneven distribution, the most common being too small a sample size.

Was the Study Double-Blinded?

If only the patient/participant is unaware of the group assignment, the study is called "single-blind"; if both participants and investigators are unaware, it is called "double-blind." A third blind can be applied to the outcome assessor (e.g., a statistician or clinician whose role is to measure the outcome). The necessity for blinding outcome assessors is controversial at this time.

～
Scenario
～

Continuing your review of weight loss interventions, you pulled this randomized crossover trial conducted in morbidly obese participants, which examined the efficacy and safety of intragastric balloon insertion. In the 1980s, researchers hypothesized that inflating a balloon in the stomach would make the individual feel full (reach satiety quicker), and therefore eat less and lose weight. The Methods section of the first randomized trial addressing the efficacy of this intervention reads:

> *A special system was designed whereby neither the patient nor the investigator could perceive the difference between sham-balloon or real balloon placement. This feat required adaptation of the existing system. Both systems were provided by the balloon manufacturer, who coded the balloon systems according to sealed coded envelopes.*
>
> *Endoscopy was performed under IV sedation with midazolam 15 mg, while the eyes of the patients were covered with a towel. After removal of the endoscope, the ready-to-use introduction system of similar design in both treatment groups was inserted up to 2 cm beyond the previously measured distance from the incisor teeth to the diaphragm. The insertion system was held in a constant position while the balloon was placed in the stomach by pushing out the balloon-loaded inner tube, audible by a click. In case of a sham procedure, the inner tube was empty. Then the air pump was connected to the inflation tube, and the balloon was inflated by five pump strokes (475 mL of room air). A quick pull at the inflation tube detached it from the one-way valve in the balloon. In case of an absent balloon (sham procedure), a resistance was built in that felt, upon inflation, the same as balloon inflation. Upon disconnection, a similar click was felt and heard...*

To minimize performance bias (systematic differences in the care provided, apart from the intervention being studied), participants and investigators must be unaware of the therapy received. Surgical procedures are often given as an example in which blinding is impossible. In the scenario, the investigators carefully designed the trial to blind not only the participants but also the surgeon. The surgeon followed the same procedures whether the participant was randomized to balloon or sham-balloon placement. The surgeon felt the same resistance at the time of inflation whether or not a balloon was attached at the end of the catheter, and heard a similar sound at the time to disconnect the balloon from the catheter, making it almost impossible for the surgeon to know to which group the participant was assigned.

User Tip

Potential breaches of blinding include using an active drug with a bitter taste and an insipid placebo, or using an active drug with significant adverse effects such as nausea and vomiting that would make it obvious to both participants and investigators which patients are receiving the active drug.

The double-blind method prevents participants or investigators from adding any additional treatments (or cointerventions) to one of the groups. For example, investigators who know that certain patients are receiving the therapy the investigators perceive to be less effective (control group; i.e., the sham-balloon placement) may opt to check on those patients more often than is required in the study protocol. The more frequent follow-up (in a weight loss trial, for example) may result in better adherence and persistence with the therapy (diet or weight loss drug) and improved outcome (better weight loss than expected from the control group). Similarly, participants who are aware of their treatment assignments may expect certain results (adverse effects or beneficial outcomes), which could influence the final end point. For example, subjects enrolled in a double-blind RCT evaluating the efficacy of *Echinacea angustifolia* roots on rhinovirus infection were asked at the end of the trial which medication they believed they were taking.[18] The volunteers who believed they were taking the active *Echinacea* had a statistically lower symptom score than the volunteers who thought they were getting a placebo.

Blinding is critical when the end point assessment can be biased by the participant or the observer (e.g., pain relief), when some other effective therapy is available and might be added to the participant's regimen, and when investigators might tend to allow participants to drop out from one therapy as they begin to suspect that the other treatment is proving to be better.

Were All Appropriate Outcomes Considered?

The first step in making any decision about initiating drug therapy is to consider the clinical value of the beneficial outcomes reported. Are the outcomes demonstrating improvements important to the patients or the question at hand? For example, a drug that has been shown to improve only left ventricular ejection fraction (surrogate marker) does not have the same clinical value as a drug that has been shown to improve hard clinical outcomes, such as decreasing mortality or improving functional status in individuals with heart failure.

~

Scenario

~

You are reviewing a head-to-head randomized trial comparing two anticoagulants to prevent venous thromboembolism (VTE) in patients undergoing hip replacement. The results are reported as follows. At day 11, the incidence of VTE was significantly reduced with drug A (4%) versus drug B (9%), leading to a relative risk reduction of 55.9% (P < .0001). In addition, the incidence of any deep venous thrombosis (DVT), proximal DVT, or distal DVT was significantly reduced with drug A (4%, 1%, and 3%, respectively) versus drug B (9%, 2%, and 7%, respectively), yielding relative risk reductions of 56.1% (P < .0001), 73.8% (P = .0021), and 54.8% (P < .0001), respectively. No difference in symptomatic VTE was observed between the groups.

Whether one drug is better than another in reducing VTE may not reflect the entire picture. First, were the DVTs detected via venography (the gold standard for research) or ultrasound (a diagnostic tool commonly used in clinical practice)? Different diagnostic methods may influence the type of patients enrolled as well as the severity or applicability of the final outcome measured. Second, is the benefit observed related to symptomatic or asymptomatic DVTs? Do asymptomatic DVTs influence prognosis? Third, is the benefit for drug A on proximal versus distal DVTs? Which outcome (proximal or distal DVT or both) is more relevant to the patient for short-term and long-term prognosis?

All these questions are quite controversial, and a clinician might pick one drug over the other depending on personal opinions. Cost and safety also must be factored into the decision. Before one regimen is adopted over another, a risk–benefit assessment is essential. The evidence must provide both efficacy and safety outcomes (mortality rate, rates of minor and major bleeding events) to make this assessment possible.

Was Intention-to-Treat Analysis Performed?

Ideally, the number of participants who entered the trial and the number of participants accounted for at the trial's conclusion are identical. Minimizing attrition bias (systematic differences in withdrawals from the trial) requires that all participants be analyzed in the groups

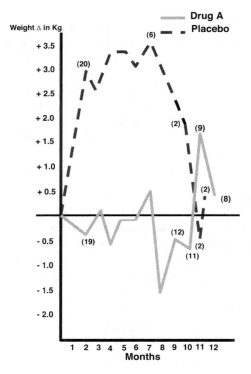

Weight Δ in Kg

Figure 3-4
The risk of withdrawal/attrition bias. Over a period of 12 months, the placebo group (*dotted line*) lost 90% of the participants originally randomized, and the treatment group lost 50%. First, using a completers analysis, rather than intention-to-treat, can be misleading. Second, a significant dropout rate such as this example makes the result difficult to interpret. (Adapted from Douglas JG, Gough J, Preston PG, et al. Long-term efficacy of fenfluramine in treatment of obesity. *Lancet.* 1983;8321:384–6, Copyright (1983), with permission from Elsevier.)

to which they were initially allocated, regardless of whether they complied with the treatment they were given. This approach is called an intention-to-treat analysis.[19]

The intention-to-treat approach has two main purposes. First, these analyses preserve the balance between treatment groups achieved by randomization. For example, in a randomized controlled trial (Figure 3-4), 42 obese women were assigned to either drug A or matching placebo, but toward the end of the study few patients remained. A completers analysis at 12 months, rather than an intent-to-treat analysis, would conclude a similar effect of placebo to drug A on weight loss. Perhaps the 18 patients in the placebo group who had dropped out had become frustrated with their lack of weight reduction, and the pair of remaining patients had both begun losing weight for other reasons. Failure to keep the last recorded weights of all patients in the data set for the balance of the study can lead to such uncertain situations.

Second, the intention-to-treat analysis is a more realistic view of how treatments will perform in actual clinical practice. In practice, patients may not adhere and persist with their medication regimens: They may change treatments along the way, or they may die before or during treatment. Also, participants may decide to drop out of the trial for many reasons (e.g., perceived treatment ineffectiveness, serious adverse effects, moving from a geographic area, loss of motivation).

When a subject withdraws before the end of treatment, the last observation (outcome measured) is carried forward to the end of treatment. The last observation carried forward (LOCF) is an analytic approach used to reduce the effect of withdrawal and still account for the subject in the final intention-to-treat analysis. Some participants will withdraw and be lost to follow-up (no outcomes available). When the percentage of patients lost to follow-up exceeds 20%, researchers and clinicians start to worry about significant withdrawal bias that may interfere with the credibility of the results. The impact of large numbers of withdrawals can be analyzed by recalculating the outcomes, assuming that all participants lost from the treatment group had the worst possible outcomes and that all participants who left the control group had the best outcomes. If this recalculation does not change the results, then regardless of the size of the withdrawal rate, the results are robust enough to be true in this worst-case scenario.

Pragmatic Versus Explanatory Analyses

Intention-to-treat analysis, by addressing the effectiveness of therapy when given to all study participants, is considered a pragmatic analysis of study data. It helps identify the utility of the treatment in clinical practice, including all patients (adherent and nonadherent, as in the real world).

Alternative analyses—including explanatory or on-drug analysis—can provide complementary information and isolate the effect of the therapy by including only participants who took the drug for a predetermined percentage of the time. Although these analyses are useful to identify the drug effect in adherent participants, their results should be used with caution in extrapolations to real-world conditions.

Assessing Validity of Systematic Reviews[20,21]

Systematic reviews that assess the results from multiple, high-quality RCTs provide the best evidence on the efficacy of drug therapy (although some would argue that mega trials provide the best evidence). Systematic reviews are valuable tools to assess generalizability and consistency or inconsistency of findings from individual RCTs. Systematic reviews can determine the consistency among studies of the same intervention (drug therapy) or whether findings from a study diverge for some reason (e.g., patients with particular risk factors, different way of measuring same outcome).

Pooling is a mathematical technique that combines results from several trials to increase sample size. Pooling the results of several RCTs yields a quantitative systematic review (most commonly called a meta-analysis). A meta-analysis provides greater statistical power and precision in estimating effects and risks than the results of any of the individual RCTs included in the review.

Figure 3–5 illustrates a forest plot (i.e., typical graphical summary of a meta-analysis). Named after the expression "you can't see the forest for the trees," the forest plot enables the reader to draw conclusions from several individual trials and get the big picture. This example combines the results of individual studies that compared the effect of thiazolidinediones versus placebo on weight in patients with type 2 diabetes. The graph displays the mean change in weight between the treatment and placebo groups (shown as squares) and the 95% CI (shown as horizontal bars) for each of the six trials. The vertical "no difference" line (or "line of no effect"), which indicates a mean difference of zero, represents the point at which there is no difference in weight change between thiazolidinedione and placebo groups. A point estimate can be a mean, a weighted difference, an odds ratio, a relative risk, or a risk difference obtained after the pooled analysis of the combined studies. By convention, a point estimate to the left of

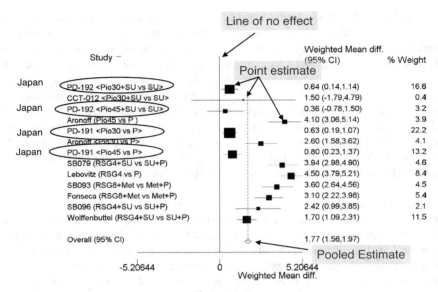

Figure 3-5

Forest plot illustrating the effect of thiazolidinediones versus placebo on weight in subjects with type 2 diabetes.

the no difference line indicates that the experimental treatment was found to provide a benefit. Likewise, a point estimate to the right of the no difference line indicates that the experimental treatment provided less benefit (more harm) than the control group. The size of the point estimate varies depending on the weight of the study. All studies are not considered equal in a meta-analysis; rather the individual studies are weighted on the basis of sample size, precision, quality, and so forth. The size of the square is proportional to the weight of the study.

When the horizontal line representing the 95% CI crosses the no difference line, the benefit or harm provided by the treatment has not reached statistical significance.

The diamond shape represents the pooled analysis. The horizontal width of the diamond corresponds to the 95% CI around the pooled estimate; the vertical corners lie on the point estimate.

In Figure 3-5, the forest plot shows a consistent weight gain with the use of thiazolidinediones except for four trials. A closer examination shows that these trials were conducted in Japan where the mean participant body mass index was less than 25 kg/m² compared with greater than 30 kg/m² for the other trials. This may explain, in part, the reason for the inconsistency in the results.

The results of systematic reviews—especially when quantified in a meta-analysis—often represent our best data about drug efficacy and safety. However, systematic reviews also should be read selectively and critically. The quality of a systematic review and its worth depend on the extent to which efforts were made to minimize error and bias.

∽

Scenario

∽

You are on rounds on the surgical ward. The attending orthopedic surgeon asks the resident whether low-molecular-weight heparins should be used before, during, or after surgery to have the best chance of preventing thrombi in a 75-year-old woman who is scheduled for elective hip replacement. The resident turns to you for an answer. You quickly browse DARE (Database of Abstracts of Reviews of Effectiveness) to see whether someone has already conducted a systematic review on the question.

Two systematic reviews published in the same journal 1 year apart reported different conclusions to the question of whether prophylaxis for venous thromboembolism with low-molecular-weight heparin should be started before or after elective hip surgery.

In the most recently published review (Hull RD, Pineo GF, Stein PD, et al. Timing of initial administration of low-molecular-weight heparin prophylaxis against deep vein thrombosis in patients following elective hip arthroplasty: a systematic review. Arch Intern Med. *2001;161:1952–60), authors concluded that delaying initiation of prophylaxis with low-molecular-weight heparin resulted in suboptimal antithrombotic effectiveness without a substantive safety advantage. This is the only systematic review reported in the DARE database. DARE includes only reviews of sufficient quality.*

In the other review (Strebel N, Prins M, Agnelli G, Buller HR. Preoperative or postoperative start of prophylaxis for venous thromboembolism with low-molecular-weight heparin in elective hip surgery? Arch Intern Med. *2002;162:1451–6), investigators reported finding no convincing evidence that starting prophylaxis preoperatively rather than postoperatively is associated with a lower incidence of venous thromboembolism.*

To formulate a response to the question at hand, the clinician first applies the screening questions to these two reviews: (1) Does each address the question? (2) Does each include the correct studies? (For a therapy question, the second question generally means that the reviews have included only RCTs.) Once both questions are answered affirmatively, each acceptable review article can then be read and critically appraised by addressing a series of concerns discussed here and summarized in the worksheet for systematic reviews provided in Appendix 3–B.

Were All Relevant Trials Found?

Just as RCTs can be biased in their inclusion of patients, systematic reviews are also at risk for selective inclusion of trials. To minimize this problem, authors of the systematic review should search several sources for eligible studies, using a comprehensive and reproducible search strategy, and also supplement their search using manual techniques of finding relevant research that might have been missed.

Search strategies should include the use of bibliographic databases (e.g., electronic databases such as MEDLINE and EMBASE), and published articles should describe the search strategy in a way that allows others to replicate the search (i.e., state the search terms, medical subject heading [MeSH] terms used, limits applied, years searched). In addition, authors should report their efforts to find additional studies that may not have been indexed by the common electronic databases or missed by the search strategy by (1) pearling (searching through the references of retrieved articles or old reviews), (2) manually searching abstracts of relevant medical conferences and journals not indexed, and (3) communicating with known experts in the field or organizations active in the area (experts may be a good source of nonpublished trials).

Were Criteria for Article Inclusion Appropriate?

The comprehensive search is likely to retrieve many articles that may not be relevant to the question at hand for a variety of reasons, including poor methodology and population differences. In the above scenario, one of the reasons for the differences between the two reviews is that they relied on differing inclusion criteria. One review included only trials that compared a low-molecular-weight heparin with warfarin, while the other included all trials of these types of heparins regardless of the comparison group.

The inclusion criteria for a systematic review should fit the four components of the well-formulated question (PICO). For example the systematic review listed in DARE included studies if they had (1) enrolled patients undergoing elective hip arthroplasty, (2) randomly assigned patients to treatment groups, (3) compared the efficacy and safety of a once-daily subcutaneous low-molecular-weight heparin with oral anticoagulants for prevention of DVT, (4) objectively documented the presence or absence of DVT using bilateral ascending contrast phlebography, and (5) used objective methods for assessing major bleeding complications.

These criteria for study inclusion fit well to the question at hand, as demonstrated by this PICO analysis:

- ≻ P: patients undergoing elective hip arthroplasty
- ≻ I: once-daily subcutaneous low-molecular-weight heparin
- ≻ C: oral anticoagulants
- ≻ O: presence or absence of DVT and proximal DVT by bilateral ascending contrast phlebography and major bleeding complications

Systematic reviews—including those that focus on a therapy question—will occasionally include trials other than randomized controlled ones. For example, authors might have selected trials that are double-blinded but not randomized or controlled, or they might include all research studies except open-label trials in which all parties (investigator, assessor, and participants) know the treatment assignment. Decisions on which trials to include in systematic reviews should be made a priori to minimize selection bias.

Was the Quality of the Individual Studies Assessed?

This criterion is a reflection of the adage "garbage in, garbage out." To combine results of RCTs that were poorly conducted—because of selection bias, errors, inadequate blinding, and other methodologic problems—will likely result in misleading conclusions.

Before including a study, the authors of a systematic review should appraise each individual study for potential bias. At a minimum, three key elements should be critically appraised: (1) adequate randomization (true randomization, with the investigator unable to predict the assigned treatment before participant entry into a trial), (2) double-blinding (masking treatment assignment to participants and investigators), and (3) control of attrition bias (all randomized participants are included in an intention-to-treat analysis).[22,23] Ideally, quality assessment should be performed by two independent reviewers to minimize selection bias.

The same process must be used if the systematic review combines results from observational studies. Each individual study should be assessed for quality by using criteria such as those listed in Appendix 3–B in the critical appraisal worksheets for various types of study methodologies.

Were Findings Combined Appropriately?

Studies sometimes produce widely divergent results when conducted similarly. In such cases, combining results to obtain an average of the treatment effect is meaningless because the average may be far from the actual results of the studies, and therefore will fail to provide accurate guidance to clinicians and researchers. Similarly, combining studies may be inappropriate if they measured different outcomes or used populations of patients that turned out to differ from one another in a perhaps unexpected way.

When the findings of individual studies are inconsistent, they should not be combined in a meta-analysis. Rather, authors of a systematic review should explore reasons why the results were so different. Questions to be asked when assessing whether the individual studies included in the systematic review were similar enough to justify combining their results in a meta-analysis include the following:

> ➤ Were the populations of the different studies similar?
> ➤ Was the same intervention evaluated by the individual studies?
> ➤ Were the same outcomes used to determine the effectiveness of the intervention being evaluated?
> ➤ Were reasons for differences among studies explored?

In short, a meta-analysis is an appropriate technique for summarizing the results of relatively homogeneous studies. It is based on the idea that the studies are sufficiently similar in their design, interventions, and participants to merit combining the data. In a meta-analysis, homogeneity can be visually assessed by displaying graphically the effect size (a way to measure the magnitude and direction of the results) or weighted means of the different trials (e.g., by using a forest plot such as that shown in Figure 3–5). As discussed above, a quick "eyeballing" of Figure 3–5 reveals that four trials are outliers; in fact, their differing results can be explained by a significant difference in the population studied (the significantly different baseline weights of the Japanese patients in the four studies and the American patients in the other trials).

A more quantitative approach for determining the appropriateness of meta-analysis is to use a statistical test of heterogeneity. This test can reveal whether the observed variability in study results (effect sizes) is greater than that expected to occur by chance. This test has low statistical power, and the boundary for statistical significance is usually set at 10%, or 0.1. A significant test means that differences exist between the individual trials and that reasons for the divergence should be explored.

What Should Be Done When Systematic Reviews Disagree?

When faced with systematic reviews with different conclusions, answering three questions can shed light on an appropriate course of action:

1. Do the reviews ask the same question?
2. Do the reviews include the same trials?
3. Is the same end point used, and are the methods of analysis comparable?

If the answer to one or more of these questions is "no," the reviews must be critically appraised to identify those most relevant to the question at hand. In some cases, one review will be more appropriate than another, but the reverse could be true with a different question.

Assessing Validity of a Cohort Study[24]

Cohort studies, also called prospective epidemiologic studies, are those in which a group of participants is identified and followed longitudinally (i.e., over a period of time) but without any overt intervention. In contrast to an RCT that seeks to compare two or more approaches to treatment, cohort studies use patients' natural demographics, lifestyles, medications, and disease histories to ferret out relationships among such factors.

Cohorts are best for prognosis types of questions, such as the following: What is the relationship between increasing cholesterol levels and heart disease? What effect on uterine cancer does use of estrogens have? Famous cohort trials include the Framingham Heart Study (ongoing information about this study is available at http://www.framingham.com/heart), Nurses' Health Study, and Physicians' Health Study.

A cohort study can also include a control group that is followed over time. For example, the link between smoking and lung disease comes from a cohort of two groups: smokers and nonsmokers. A cohort study differs from a case–control study (discussed in the next section) in that the latter is generally a retrospective analysis comparing people who already have a disease or condition (cases) with people with similar demographic and clinic characteristics who do not have the disease (controls).

⌒ *Scenario* ⌒

You are a pharmacist working in a family practice setting. One of your patients is a 30-year-old woman who has been taking oral contraceptives for the past 4 years. She calls you to say that she is concerned about taking her new birth control pills because recently she read in magazines and heard from friends that these agents may increase her risk for developing DVT. Her mom was just diagnosed with a DVT and is now on long-term warfarin prophylaxis.

For ethical and methodologic reasons, safety trials are generally not conducted by using randomized controlled research designs. However, there may be a cohort study in which women exposed to the newer oral contraceptives were followed and compared with a "similar" group of women exposed to the older class of oral contraceptives to determine the incidence of venous thromboembolism. Cohort studies are useful for harmful outcomes that are infrequent (e.g., cigarette smoking and cancer, gastrointestinal bleeds and the use of nonsteroidal anti-inflammatory drugs).

Was Recruitment Adequate?

Selection, or membership, bias related to recruitment can confound the results of a cohort study. Because the decision about who receives treatment is not randomized, exposed patients may differ from nonexposed patients with respect to important risk factors known to influence the outcome. As discussed in the section Randomization, these risk factors are called confounders, and this type of problem is called confounding bias.

Regarding the above patient, the newer oral contraceptives may be preferentially prescribed to women at risk for cardiovascular disease (prone to thrombosis) and, therefore, differ significantly from patients prescribed the older class of agents.

Several other recruitment-related questions are relevant. Are all participants at the same time point in their disease or exposure? Age, duration of treatment/exposure, and severity of the disease are all variables that can affect risk for the outcome being studied.

Where were participants recruited? A study on asthma recruiting from a pulmonology setting versus family practice will invariably recruit participants with more severe asthma.

In published studies, authors should be explicit about the baseline characteristics of both groups and describe statistical techniques later used to adjust for known confounders. In a cohort design, authors can adjust for only known confounders; unlike randomized trials, observational design does not control for unknown confounders.

Was Outcome Accurately Measured/Detected?

Surveillance bias—systematic differences in diagnosing an outcome based on heavier surveillance in the group exposed to the risk factor—can distort the outcome assessment in cohort studies. For instance, when investigators are aware that patients have been exposed to a risk factor, they have a tendency to be more diligent in their assessments (e.g., blood glucose levels are more likely to be checked in patients prescribed antipsychotic agents, increasing the probability that elevated levels will be detected). In cohort studies, this bias can be minimized by blinding the investigators doing assessments to the exposure status of patients.

The sources of cohort outcome data may vary significantly and affect the results. Morbidity and mortality data may be obtained from physicians, hospital records, medical examinations, health plan records, or questionnaires. Relative to the risk factor and outcomes being studied, some of these methods may be more sensitive than others, and the reader must consider this effect when interpreting results of cohort studies.

Was Follow-Up Long Enough?

If the clinician is interested in the long-term prognosis for patients with a disorder such as diabetes, then a study with 6 months of follow-up will probably not be very useful. In general, follow-up needs to continue long enough to make it likely that a high proportion of the participants who are going to experience a particular clinically relevant event will have done so.

Just as in controlled trials, participants sometimes drop out of cohort studies. Reasons for dropouts in each group should be assessed. For example, people who are healthier may move from an area at a greater rate and thereby be lost to follow-up; a cohort study excluding dropouts might produce an unrealistically negative outcome.

Assessing Validity of a Case–Control Study

If an outcome of interest is rare or requires a long time to develop, then case–control studies are the most efficient research design. These studies involve identifying patients who have the outcome of interest (cases) and control patients without the same outcome, and looking back to see if both groups had the exposure of interest.

Using a case–control design, investigators demonstrated an association between diethylstilbestrol (DES) ingestion by pregnant women and the development of vaginal adenocarcinoma in their daughters when they reached maturity many years later. A prospective cohort study designed to test this association would have required at least 20 years. Further, given the infrequency of the disease, a cohort study would have required hundreds of thousands of participants. Using the case–control strategy, the investigators defined two groups of women—those who had vaginal adenocarcinoma (defined as cases) and those who did not have the outcome (defined as controls) but had similar characteristics as the cases (usually controls are matched for known risk factors). The groups were then compared for their exposure or lack of exposure to DES (exposure in this case was *in utero*), and the relationship was observed.

Did Exposure Occur Before the Outcome?

The association of increased suicidal ideation with the use of antidepressants illustrates the importance of this question when case–control studies are analyzed. Did the thoughts of suicide occur more frequently after antidepressant therapy was started or the dose increased, or was therapy begun or changed because patients' depression was worsening?

Was the Control Group Well Matched?

The most critical issue with case–control studies is often the selection of a control group. When confounding factors cannot be controlled by randomization, cases (individuals with the harmful outcome) are matched with controls who have similar characteristics, such as age, to attempt to reduce the effect of the confounding factors on the association being investigated. Unknown risk factors/confounders can never be entirely corrected for in a case–control design.

Was Exposure Ascertained Adequately?

Recall bias is frequent in case–control designs. Case–control designs are commonly used to investigate teratogenic effects of drugs during pregnancy; information about drug intake is recalled by the mothers after having given birth. However, a mother who just gave birth to a child with severe or visible congenital abnormalities may be more likely to remember/recall her drug use during pregnancy than a woman who just gave birth to a healthy baby. Did the authors use other techniques or resources (e.g., pharmacy records, medical records) beyond recall to ascertain the exposure?

Case Reports and Case Series[25]

Scenario

A physician notices that two newborn babies in his hospital have absent limbs (phocomelia). Both mothers had taken a new drug (thalidomide) in early pregnancy. The physician wishes to alert his colleagues worldwide to the possibility of drug-related damage as quickly as possible. He publishes a case series reporting the two birth defects.

The anecdotal case report is at the bottom of the evidence ladder (Figure 3–1) because it provides isolated observations that are collected in an uncontrolled, unsystematic manner. When several similar cases occur, authors will describe them in a case series, but case series also present information collected in an uncontrolled manner.

The case report/case series design does not control for confounders or potential bias. Although case reports are inadequate for assessing risk or making causal associations, they have served important roles in identification of adverse effects and even unlabeled uses of medications. Case reports or systematic reviews of case reports may also be the only sources of evidence to answer questions about potential drug–drug interactions and rare adverse events. (A systematic review of case reports implies that the authors have conducted a comprehensive search of the literature using a reproducible search strategy and have summarized the findings using explicit methodology.) When these reports are the only evidence, then they are the best available evidence.

⁓
Scenario
⁓

JB, a 68-year-old married man with type 2 diabetes and known coronary heart disease, died of myocardial infarction after taking sildenafil (Viagra—Pfizer Inc.). He took the drug for erectile dysfunction and experienced chest pain after 15 minutes of intercourse with his girlfriend. JB took sublingual nitroglycerine for relief and then went home, where he died within 2 hours.

Several confounders complicate the association between phosphodiesterase type 5 inhibitors and cardiovascular death: (1) Most men with erectile dysfunction have known risk factors for increased cardiovascular death (diabetes, known coronary heart disease, age); (2) patients' cardiac workload is increased by sexual activity; (3) these agents are now known to enhance the vasodilatory effects of nitroglycerin, making combination therapy contraindicated; and (4) as in this case, a surprising number of patients experiencing the cardiac problems after use of these drugs were having sexual relations outside marriage and may have felt guilty about their actions.

Did Exposure Occur Before the Harmful Outcome?

In case reports, could the patient have had the outcome before the exposure to the drug? An outcome that takes years to develop and be diagnosed (e.g., cancer) may be present before the use of the drug, and any association between the drug and the outcome may be erroneous. The temporal relationship between drug exposure and the outcome can substantially strengthen a causal association, as in the case of anaphylaxis occurring immediately after intravenous penicillin use.

Alternatively the timing of the adverse event may be misleading. For example, liver dysfunction may manifest weeks after kava kava administration, and clinicians typically will not associate herbal use with the adverse effect.

What Happened During Dechallenge or Rechallenge?

The temporal relationship between drug exposure and the adverse effect is further strengthened when the effect disappears after the drug is stopped (dechallenge), especially if it recurs when the drug is readministered (rechallenge). Rechallenge is not always possible or ethical to conduct, but recurrence on rechallenge is strongly suggestive that the drug was responsible for observed effect.

Were Results Plausible Relative to Existing Knowledge?

Ideally, drug effects on biological systems mesh well with known facts about the medication and human physiology. For example, a recently marketed drug is reported to cause high blood pressure in a patient. But the drug, orlistat (Xenical—Hoffman-La Roche), is used for weight loss because it inhibits lipase locally in the gastrointestinal tract and is not appreciably absorbed into the bloodstream. None of the drug's biological actions or the physiology of the gastrointestinal tract readily explain the adverse event reported.

In contrast, rosiglitazone (Avandia—GlaxoSmithKline) is a peroxisome proliferator–activated receptor (PPAR) gamma agonist and was reported to exacerbate congestive heart failure. The effect could be explained by the edema known to occur with PPAR gamma agonists, offering a plausible physiologic understanding of the adverse event reported.

Table 3–3   World Health Organization Classification of Causality for Reports of Harmful Events

Causality Term	Assessment Criteria
Certain	≻ Harmful events with plausible time relationship to drug intake ≻ Harmful events cannot be explained by disease or other drugs ≻ Response to withdrawal plausible on the basis of known pharmacologic or pathologic data ≻ Harmful events reproduced at rechallenge
Probable/likely	≻ Harmful event with reasonable time relationship to drug intake ≻ Harmful event unlikely to be attributed to disease or other drugs ≻ Response to withdrawal clinically reasonable ≻ Rechallenge not required
Possible	≻ Harmful events with reasonable time relationship to drug intake ≻ Harmful events could also be explained by disease or other drugs ≻ Information on drug withdrawal may be lacking or unclear
Unlikely	≻ Harmful events with a time to drug intake that makes a relationship improbable (but not impossible) ≻ Disease or other drugs provide plausible explanations
Unassessable/unclassifiable	≻ Adverse reaction suggested in a report ≻ Harmful event cannot be judged because information is insufficient or contradictory ≻ Data cannot be supplemented or verified

Source: Adapted from information on World Health Organization Web site. Information can be found at http://www.who-umc.org/DynPage.aspx?id=22682.

Was There a Dose–Response Relationship?

The majority of adverse reactions reported are idiosyncratic and are not dose related. Examples of such reactions are rash with penicillins and thrombocytopenia with clopidogrel (Plavix—Bristol-Myers Squibb). However, adverse events associated with the primary pharmacologic effect of the drug or those caused by its other effects are dose related, and typically appear or worsen with a dose increase and abate with dosage reduction. Ototoxicity and nephrotoxicity with aminoglycosides, respiratory failure with morphine, and nausea with glucagon-like peptide-1 are examples of these effects. Presence of a dose–response relationship strengthens the association between drug exposure and drug effect.

Were the Results Consistent with Previous Reports?

Is this a single report, or is the effect being reported by others describing similar circumstances and outcomes? Depending on the quality, completeness, and seriousness of the adverse event, a single report may be sufficient to raise concerns, but generally several cases consistently reporting an association are needed.

Was There Causality?

Table 3–3 describes the criteria developed by the World Health Organization to define causality. A "probable" causal association is considered to be one in which the time sequence is reasonable, the event is unlikely to be attributable to concurrent disease or other medicines, and a clinically reasonable response follows withdrawal. Rechallenge information is not essential to fulfill the definition. A "possible" causality assessment also requires a reasonable time sequence, but the event may also be explained by concurrent disease or other medicines, and information on withdrawal may be lacking or unclear.

Grading Recommendations According to the Evidence Ladder

Dozens of different classification schemes are available for grading recommendations on the basis of evidence (the CD provided with this book has examples of different classifications). The Agency for Healthcare Research and Quality has identified three key elements that should be part of the grading system: quality, certainty, and consistency.[26] The rating system should be based on the quality of the individual studies on which the recommendation is based. The quality assessment refers to the internal validity of the individual trials. A quality scale, such as the Jadad quality scale (most popular scale) at http://www.uea.ac.uk/~wp276/moher.htm, or the critical appraisal checklists in Appendix 3–B can be used to ensure that the conduct of the trial minimized bias. The certainty of the trial depends on the size, power, and magnitude of the beneficial or harmful effect. Finally, findings should be replicated in several RCTs or studies using other reliable designs.

The most commonly used classification is from the Centre for Evidence-Based Medicine (available at http://www.cebm.net/levels_of_evidence.asp). The rating system has two layers: the individual evidence is rated (level 1 to 5) on the basis of the quality/internal validity and certainty of its results, and the recommendation/statement based on the evidence is graded (A to D) depending on the level of evidence supporting it.

The Bottom Line

➢ Do not believe everything you read.

➢ Answer these two questions:
  —Does the study clearly define the question and is it pertinent to my question?
  —Does the study design match my question?
  —If the answer is "yes" to both, read beyond the abstract.

➢ These primary questions apply to all study types:
  —Is the comparison group identical in all aspects other than the intervention or exposure?
  —Are management and outcome assessment the same in all groups?
  —Are all participants accounted for?

➢ Access to critical appraisal worksheets is available at these Web sites:
  —Critical Appraisal Skill Programme:
    http://www.pdptoolkit.co.uk/Files/ebm/indexes/guide%20to%20ebm.htm.
  —Centre for Evidence-Based Medicine: http://www.cebm.net/downloads.asp.

References

1. Smith GC, Pell JP. Parachute use to prevent death and major trauma related to gravitational challenge: systematic review of randomised controlled trials. *BMJ*. 2003;327(7429):1459–61.

2. Echt DS, Liebson PR, Mitchell B, et al. Mortality and morbidity in patients receiving encainide, flecainide or placebo: The Cardiac Arrhythmia Suppression Trial. *N Engl J Med*. 1991;324:781–8.

3. Greene HL, Roden DM, Katz RJ, et al. The Cardiac Arrhythmia Suppression Trial: First CAST, then CAST-II. *J Am Coll Cardiol*. 1992;19:894–8.

4. Antman EM, Anbe DT, Armstrong PW, et al. ACC/AHA Guidelines for the Management of patients with ST-elevation myocardial infarction—executive summary: A report of the American College of Cardiology/American Heart Association Task Force on Practice Guidelines (Writing Committee to Revise the 1999 Guidelines for the Management of Patients With Acute Myocardial Infarction). *Circulation*. 2004;110:588–636.

5. Ryan TJ, Anderson JL, Antman EM, et al. ACC/AHA guidelines for the management of patients with acute myocardial infarction: A report of the American College of Cardiology/American Heart Association Task Force on Practice Guidelines (Committee on Management of Acute Myocardial Infarction). *J Am Coll Cardiol*. 1996;28:1328–428.

6. Hulley S, Grady D, Bush T, et al, for the Heart and Estrogen/progestin Replacement Study (HERS) Research Group. Randomized trial of estrogen plus progestin for secondary prevention of coronary heart disease in postmenopausal women. *JAMA*. 1998;280:605–13.

7. Rossouw JE, Anderson GL, Prentice RL, et al., for the Writing Group for the Women's Health Initiative Investigators. Risks and benefits of estrogen plus progestin in healthy postmenopausal women: principal results from the Women's Health Initiative randomized controlled trial. *JAMA*. 2002;288(3):321–33. PMID: 12117397.

8. Grady D, Herrington D, Bittner V, et al, for the HERS Research Group. Cardiovascular disease outcomes during 6.8 years of hormone therapy: Heart and Estrogen/progestin Replacement Study follow-up (HERS II). *JAMA*. 2002;288:49–57.

9. LeLorier J, Gregorie G, Benhaddad A, et al. Discrepancies between meta-analyses and subsequent large randomised controlled trials. *N Engl J Med*. 1997;337:536–42.

10. Egger M, Davey Smith G, Schneider M, Minder C. Bias in meta-analysis detected by a simple, graphical test. *BMJ*. 1997;315(7109):629–34.

11. Teo KK, Yusuf S, Collins R, et al. Effects of intravenous magnesium in suspected acute myocardial infarction: overview of randomised trials. *BMJ*. 1991;303:1499–1503.

12. ISIS-4 (Fourth International Study of Infarct Survival) Collaborative Group. ISIS-4: a randomised factorial trial assessing early oral captopril, oral mononitrate, and intravenous magnesium sulphate in 58050 patients with suspected acute myocardial infarction. *Lancet*. 1995;345:669–85.

13. Villar J, Carroli G, Belizan JM. Predictive ability of meta-analyses of randomised controlled trials. *Lancet*. 1995;345:772–6.

14. Cappelleri JC, Ioannidis JPA, Schmid CH, et al. Large trials vs meta-analysis of smaller trials. How do their results compare? *JAMA*. 1996;276:1332–8.

15. Guyatt G, Sackett D, Cook D. Users' guides to the medical literature, II. How to use an article about therapy or prevention. A. Are the results of the study valid? Evidence-Based Medicine Working Group. *JAMA*. 1993;270(21):2598–601.

16. Emerson JD, Burdick E, Hoaglin DC, et al. An empirical study of the possible relation of treatment differences to quality scores in controlled randomized clinical trials. *Control Clin Trials*. 1990;11:339–52.

17. Chalmers TC, Celano P, Sacks HS, Smith H Jr. Bias in treatment assignment in controlled clinical trials. *N Engl J Med*. 1983;309:1358–61.

18. Turner RB, Bauer R, Woelkart K, et al. An evaluation of Echinacea angustifolia in experimental rhinovirus infections. *N Engl J Med*. 2005;353:341–8.

19. Hollis S, Campbell F. What is meant by intention to treat analysis? Survey of published randomised controlled trials. *BMJ*. 1999;319:670–4.

20. Oxman AD, Cook DJ, Guyatt GH. Users' guides to the medical literature, VI. How to use an overview. Evidence-Based Medicine Working Group. *JAMA*. 1994;272(17):1367–71.

21. Oxman AD. Checklists for review articles. *BMJ*. 1994;309:648–51.

22. Moher D, Jadad AR, Nichol G, et al. Assessing the quality of randomized controlled trials: an annotated bibliography of scales and checklists. *Control Clin Trials*. 1995;16(1):62–73.

23. Jadad AR, Moore RA, Carrol D, et al. Assessing the quality of reports of randomized clinical trials: is blinding necessary? *Control Clin Trials*. 1996;17:1–12.

24. Laupacis A, Wells G, Richardson WS, Tugwell P. Users' guides to the medical literature, V. How to use an article about prognosis. Evidence-Based Medicine Working Group. *JAMA*. 1994;272(3):234–7.

25. Naranjo CA, Busto U, Sellers EM, et al. A method for estimating the probability of adverse drug reactions. *Clin Pharmacol Ther*. 1981;30:239–45.

26. Systems to rate the strength of scientific evidence. Summary, evidence report/technology assessment: number 47. AHRQ publication no. 02-E015, March 2002. Rockville, Md: Agency for Healthcare Research and Quality. Available at: http://www.ahrq.gov/clinic/epcsums/strenfact.htm. Accessed October 13, 2006.

APPENDIX 3–A
BASIC DESIGNS OF CLINICAL RESEARCH

Clinical research can be experimental or observational. In experimental studies, an intervention (drug or procedure) is performed under the control of the investigator. In observational studies, the investigator observes patients at a point in time (cross-sectional studies) or over time (longitudinal studies). One or more groups are observed and outcomes are recorded. If the observations are made by looking forward and gathering new data, the study is prospective; if the outcome already occurred (e.g., the investigator reviews medical records or a pharmacy database to collect the outcome), the study is retrospective.

Observational Study Designs

Case Reports and Case Series

A case report provides a descriptive summary of observations from one patient, while a case series provides a descriptive summary of observations from a group of people with the same condition (Figure A3–1). These study designs are often used to describe a generally rare adverse event (e.g., rhabdomyolysis with rosuvastatin [Crestor—Astra-Zeneca Pharmaceuticals]) of a new therapy, a new indication for an old therapy (e.g., tricyclic antidepressants to reduce neuropathic pain), or the management of a rare disorder. They often provide valuable information that cannot be found in clinical trials. Case reports have been crucial to alert the world to important health risks or health benefits associated with new therapies. For example, cases of valvulopathy with the use of fenfluramine (Pondimin—Wyeth-Ayerst Laboratories) were first reported as case reports and resulted in the withdrawal of the weight loss drug. A case report can provide the basis for a hypothesis, which can be studied in a more rigorous trial.

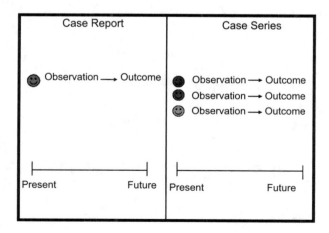

Figure A3-1
Case report/case series design schematic.

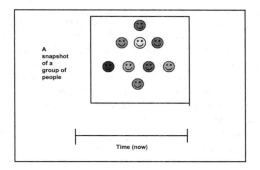

Figure A3-2
Cross-sectional design schematic.

Despite the important role these studies can play, they are found at the bottom of the evidence ladder, because they represent isolated observations that are collected in an uncontrolled, unsystematic manner.

Examples of questions that best match a case report/case-series include the following:

➢ Is there any report of agranulocytosis with losartan (Cozaar—Merck & Co., Inc.)?
➢ Is there any report of using enoxaparin (Lovenox—sanofi-aventis) to prevent post-stent thrombosis?

Cross-Sectional Study

A cross-sectional study (also called prevalence survey) can be thought of as providing a "snapshot" of a group of people at a single point in time or over a short period of time (Figure A3-2). For instance, a large cross-section of women with breast cancer might be interviewed to determine their hygiene habits such as the use of antiperspirants. Although this type of study is relatively easy and inexpensive to carry out, it can establish only an association, not a cause-and-effect relationship. The design is susceptible to recall bias, which occurs when participants in one group are more likely to remember/recall the event than those in the other group. For example, a patient who just suffered a stroke is more likely to remember events (e.g., what they ate the night of the stroke, medications they were on) at the time in question than would a healthy patient. Because exposure and disease status are measured at the same point in time, it may not always be possible to distinguish whether the exposure preceded or followed the disease (the chicken-or-egg phenomenon) as illustrated by the following questions: Are patients with peptic ulcer drinking more milk because of their peptic ulcer, or is drinking more milk causing peptic ulcer?

Some questions that best match a cross-sectional study include the following:

➢ What is the prevalence of obesity in the United States?
➢ How many new hospital admissions are caused by medication misuse?
➢ Is there an association between cleft palate and the use of Bendectin (doxylamine/ dicyclomine/pyridoxine—Merrel Dow Pharmaceuticals; drug voluntarily removed from market) during pregnancy?

Case–Control Study

In this type of study, people with a particular condition (cases) are matched with a group of people who do not have the disorder (controls). (The cases have the disease; the controls do not have the disease but are matched to have similar characteristics, such as age, gender, and risk factors, so that they are similar to the cases in all relevant ways except for presence of the disease.) The researchers look back in time to determine the proportion of people in each group who were exposed to the suspected causal factor (Figure A3–3). This study is relatively quick and inexpensive, and is often the best design for rare disorders or disorders with a long time lag between the exposure and the outcome.

The major disadvantage of this type of study is that it relies on memory (recall bias) or on medical records, which may be inaccurate or incomplete. Selection bias is also likely in case–control studies. For example, the cases may be more likely to be exposed to the drug because of

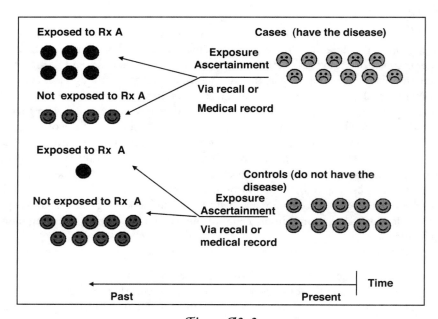

Figure A3–3
Case–control design schematic.

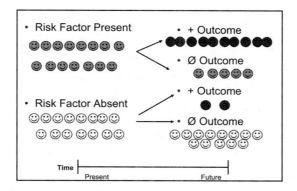

Figure A3–4
Cohort design schematic.

the severity of their disease or because of socioeconomic status, resulting in selection bias. As mentioned earlier with respect to hormone-replacement therapy, case–control study findings should be confirmed with a randomized controlled trial.

Examples of questions that best match a case–control study include the following:

➤ Do selective serotonin reuptake inhibitors increase the risk of suicide?
➤ Are calcium channel blockers associated with an increased risk of cancer?
➤ Can rofecoxib (Vioxx—Merck & Co., Inc.) increase the risk of myocardial infarction?

Cohort Study

A major limitation of cross-sectional and case-control studies is the difficulty in determining whether the risk factor (or exposure) was present before the disease. In contrast, the cohort study design follows a group of subjects over time and can control for the presence or absence of risk factors before the outcome occurs (Figure A3–4). Because the cohort follows people over time, these studies have the appropriate time sequence to ascertain a possible cause-and-effect relationship.

The Framingham Heart Study is perhaps the best-known research effort that used a cohort design. The original enrollees, 5209 men and women aged 28 to 62 years who lived in the Boston suburb of Framingham, Massachusetts, entered the study from 1948 to 1952. Participants have been examined every 2 years since that time, and the cohort has been followed for morbidity and mortality. The study has identified critical risk factors for arteriosclerosis and played a pivotal role in the current risk assessment classification for coronary artery disease. The National Heart, Lung, and Blood Institute provides ongoing information about this study at http://www.framingham.com/heart.

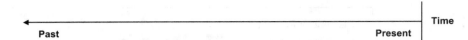

Figure A3–5
Historical/retrospective cohort schematic.

Variations of the Cohort Design

Historical/Retrospective   As shown in Figure A3–5, in a historical/retrospective design, outcomes have already occurred and researchers are looking back through medical records.

Nested Case–Control   This variation is a case–control analysis performed within a cohort. For example, during the follow-up of the cohort, some people develop the disease, while others remain disease-free. The cases (participants who have the disease) are compared with the controls (participants who are disease-free) within the same cohort, and researchers look back to determine exposure to a drug or other factor.
    The following questions best match a cohort:

 ➢ Are people with elevated cholesterol at increased risk for coronary artery disease?
 ➢ Are obese people at increased risk for degenerative joint disease?
 ➢ Are people with hepatitis C more likely to develop liver cancer?

Experimental Studies or Clinical Trial Designs

Experimental studies can be either controlled (there is a comparison group) or uncontrolled. Uncontrolled studies provide weak evidence and should be considered as observational. These studies could be useful early in drug development to explore safety or generate baseline data to help plan future controlled trials, but not to guide practice. The experimental designs enable the investigators to draw conclusions about causes and relationships, a process that is not possible with observational designs. The purpose of the experimental design is to establish the real effect of the intervention (drug) and rule out other causes for the effect observed.

Randomized Controlled Trials

Randomized trials are the gold standard for questions specific to the efficacy and/or safety of a drug therapy. Randomization minimizes the risk that unknown confounders are distributed unequally between groups. A randomized trial means that the participants had an equal chance to be assigned to group A or group B (Figure A3–6).
    Examples of questions best answered by randomized controlled trials include the following:

 ➢ Is drug X better than or equal to drug Y to prevent disease?
 ➢ Is drug X better than or equal to drug Y to treat disease?
 ➢ Is drug X better than or equal to placebo to prevent disease?
 ➢ Is drug X better than or equal to placebo to treat disease?
 ➢ Is a certain intervention (e.g., surgery, diet, exercise) better than or equal to drug X (or another intervention) for treating (or preventing) disease?

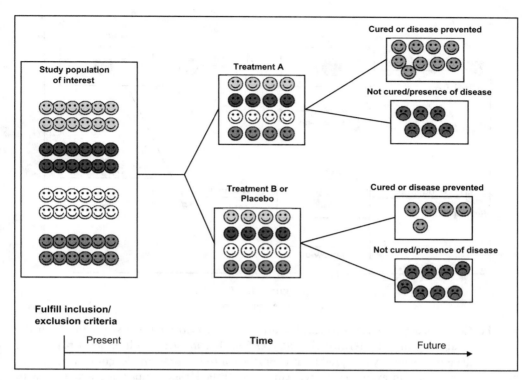

Figure A3-6
Randomized trial design schematic.

Variations of the Randomized Trial

Crossover Study   In a crossover design, all participants are randomized to a sequence of treatments. For example, participant 1 is randomized to drug A first, then crossed over to drug B, while participant 2 is randomized to drug B first then crossed over to drug A (Figure A3–7). Thus, participants are given two or more treatments in sequence. Crossover designs are very commonly used in pharmacokinetic studies in which two or more formulations of a drug are assessed for bioequivalence.

Because each participant in a crossover study serves as his or her own control, this design is more efficient than a parallel group type of design, thus allowing smaller sample size. However, crossover designs carry sources of bias, referred to as "treatment period interaction." Because of the possibility that carryover effects from the first period may carry over into subsequent periods (i.e., effects of the first treatment may still be present for a long period, or the first treatment permanently changes the course of the disease), crossover trials cannot be used for certain types of treatment comparisons. Also, responses in the second treatment period may differ from those in the first period. For example, receptors may still be occupied by the drug from the first period or may have been upregulated by the effect of the drug on the first period, the disease severity may have changed in the second treatment period, or other patient-specific circumstances may have caused the patient to respond differently.

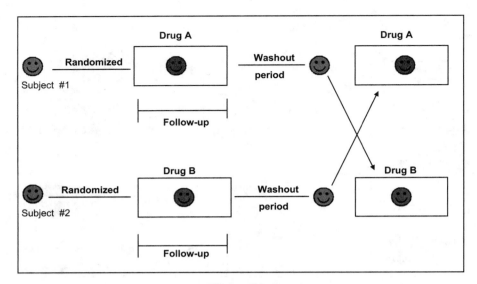

Figure A3-7
Crossover design schematic.

Placebo-Controlled Versus Head-to-Head Study   A controlled trial is a study in which the experimental drug (usually termed the *intervention*) is compared with either a placebo or another drug or previously accepted treatment (the *control*). For example, comparing enoxaparin (Lovenox—sanofi-aventis) with heparin is a controlled trial, comparing enoxaparin with placebo is a controlled trial, and comparing orlistat (Xenical—Hoffman-La Roche) with usual care of obesity is also a controlled trial.

Use of placebo controls in a clinical trial can be unethical. If a generally accepted treatment can improve survival or morbidity of the population being studied, then an active control is preferred over placebo.

Head-to-head controlled trials are those that compare drugs within a pharmacologic class (e.g., pravastatin [various manufacturers] versus atorvastatin [Lipitor—Pfizer Inc.]) or indicated for the disease under study (e.g., angiotensin-converting enzyme inhibitors versus thiazides for treatment of hypertension) with the objective to determine whether differences exist in safety or efficacy between or among the drugs.

Factorial Designs   Most experimental designs ask what is the effect of intervention A on outcome X. But at times one may want to know the effect of intervention A or B combined with drug C or D on one outcome. For example, the Bypass Angioplasty Revascularization Investigation (BARI) 2D trial is a multicenter study that uses a 2 × 2 factorial design (Figure A3–8). The 2800 patients with diabetes and chest pain were assigned at random to initial elective revascularization with aggressive medical therapy or to aggressive medical therapy alone with equal probability. In addition, they were assigned simultaneously at random to an insulin-providing or insulin-sensitizing strategy for glycemic control. In other words, the patient with diabetes and chest pain enrolled in BARI 2D is randomized to one of four interventions: catheterization plus a thiazolidinedione, catheterization plus insulin or insulin secretagogue, aggressive medical therapy (but no catheterization) plus a thiazolidinedione, or aggressive medical therapy plus insulin or insulin secretagogues.

Figure A3–9 illustrates a 3 × 2 factorial design.

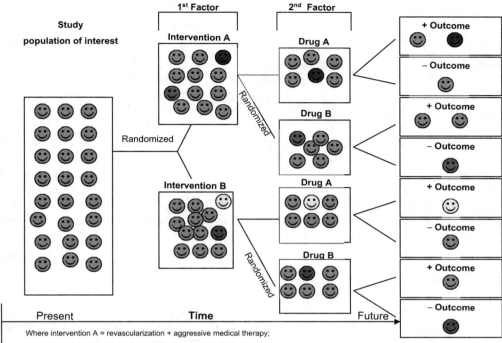

Where intervention A = revascularization + aggressive medical therapy;

intervention B = aggressive medical therapy without revascularization.

Drug A = insulin-providing strategy to control glycemia.

Drug B = insulin-sensitization strategy to control glycemia.

Figure A3–8

2 × 2 factorial design schematic.

	Vitamin	Placebo
Drug A	Drug A + Vitamin	Drug A + Placebo
Drug B	Drug B + Vitamin	Drug B + Placebo
Drug C	Drug C + Vitamin	Drug C + Placebo

Figure A3–9

3 × 2 factorial design schematic.

Block Designs: Stratified Strategies "Block what you can, randomize what you cannot" is the underlying principle in studies that use block designs. Blocking is used when the investigator is aware of specific characteristics or risk factors known to affect clinical outcomes in patients with the disease in question. If, for instance, investigators believe that age may affect patients' response to a drug, they might choose to first divide the participants into age groups (e.g., younger than 40 years, between 40 and 65 years old, and older than 65 years). Participants are then randomized within each block of age. The block design is an attempt at controlling a known confounder.

Equivalence Versus Noninferiority Trial Designs   The objective of equivalence trials is to determine whether the experimental drug is similar to an active control treatment. For instance, bioequivalence studies comparing generic drugs with brand-name innovator products are true equivalence trials. The effects of the generic drug should not differ by more than the amount established a priori—the equivalence margin—on both sides of the values for half-life, peak and/or trough concentrations, and areas under the serum concentration–time curves.

The objective of noninferiority trials is to demonstrate whether the experimental drug is no worse than an active control. This is a one-sided research question because the investigators are interested only in whether the experimental drug has decreased efficacy by an equivalence margin defined a priori. These trials do not consider safety; therefore, when interpreting their results, clinicians must keep in mind that two drugs may be equivalent in efficacy, but have significant differences in their adverse effect profiles.

Systematic Reviews and Meta-Analyses

A systematic review is a comprehensive review article that summarizes and/or describes a collection of quality trials (most commonly randomized controlled trials) addressing a similar question with the purpose of drawing general conclusions. In contrast to a narrative review article, the systematic review follows a rigorous methodology to minimize bias in all parts of its process: identification and selection of trials, data collection, and pooling of the data. Other elements that distinguish systematic reviews from traditional narrative reviews include the scope of the review. Systematic reviews are generated to answer in-depth, specific, and often narrow clinical questions. Most narrative review articles deal with a broad range of issues related to a given topic rather than a particular issue in depth.

Systematic reviews use a comprehensive, reproducible data search, and follow a rigorous selection and abstraction process that is described in advance. Traditional narrative reviews most often include a subset of all relevant references.

Systematic reviews follow a standard process to critically appraise data, while traditional reviews do not explicitly describe their processes for critically appraising the selected literature.

Finally, traditional reviews summarize their data qualitatively. Systematic reviews, when feasible, use quantitative methods and thereby provide estimates of treatment effects or exposure risks. When the systematic review performs such a quantitative analysis, it is referred to as a meta-analysis. In a systematic review the unit of analysis is the primary study (Figure A3–10).

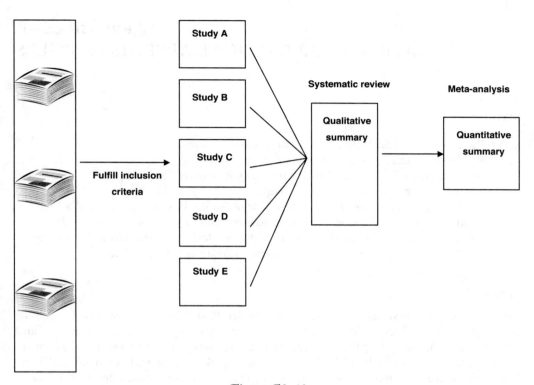

Figure A3–10
Systematic review/meta-analysis design schematic.

APPENDIX 3–B
APPLY YOUR CRITICAL APPRAISAL SKILLS

Web Tutorials

> ➤ The University of Sheffield tutorial with worked examples:
> http://www.shef.ac.uk/scharr/ir/units/critapp.
> ➤ Centre for Evidence-Based Medicine tutorial with worked examples:
> —http://www.cebm.utoronto.ca/practise/ca.
> ➤ The Michigan State University, Department of Family Practice, has created a Web-based tutorial that introduces the basic concepts of information mastery, evidence-based medicine, and critical appraisal of the medical literature. Work the therapy case: http://www.poems.msu.edu/infomastery/Treatment/treatment.htm.

Scenario 1

You are a hospital pharmacist practicing in October 2004. The cyclooxygenase-2 inhibitor rofecoxib (Vioxx—Merck & Co. Inc.) has just been removed from the market worldwide, and all product in your hospital has been returned to the manufacturer. A patient who has not yet discontinued Vioxx is admitted. The floor nurse calls to ask you what we have to replace Vioxx. The doctor suggested naproxen as a replacement. The nurse is concerned whether it will be as good for pain relief. You formulate the question: In this 65-year-old man with osteoarthritis, is naproxen as safe (to avoid gastrointestinal bleed) and effective (for pain control) as rofecoxib? You search PubMed for a head-to-head randomized controlled trial that may give you a sense of the efficacy and safety profile of naproxen compared with Vioxx. You find the article Lisse JR, Perlman M, Johansson G, et al. Gastrointestinal tolerability and effectiveness of rofecoxib versus naproxen in the treatment of osteoarthritis: a randomized, controlled trial. *Ann Intern Med.* 2003;139(7):539–46.

Read the article and formulate a recommendation as to whether the patient should be switched to naproxen. For your analysis, use the appropriate critical appraisal worksheet for randomized controlled trials provided as a tool at the end of this appendix.

Scenario 2

You are on rounds in the surgical ward. The attending orthopedic surgeon asks the resident whether low-molecular-weight heparins should be used before, during, or after surgery to prevent thromboprophylaxis in a 75-year-old woman scheduled for elective hip replacement. The resident turns to you for an answer. You quickly browse DARE (Database of Abstracts of Reviews of Effectiveness) to see whether someone has already done a systematic review on the question. You find two systematic reviews: (1) Strebel N, Prins M, Agnelli G, et al. Preoperative or postoperative start of prophylaxis for venous thromboembolism with low-molecular-weight heparin in elective hip surgery? *Arch Intern Med.* 2002;162:1451–6 and (2) Hull R, Pineo G, Stein P, et al. Timing of initial administration of low-molecular-weight heparin prophylaxis against deep vein thrombosis in patients following elective hip arthroplasty. *Arch Intern Med.* 2001;161:1952–60.

Read both systematic reviews and decide which one has the correct conclusion. Use the appropriate critical appraisal worksheet for systematic reviews provided at the end of this appendix.

Scenario 3

A patient asks your advice on whether she should buy glucosamine/chondroitin to reduce her joint pain. She says that her physician told her to take acetaminophen for her osteoarthritis. She read and several friends told her that the combination of glucosamine and chondroitin could improve her walking. Is it true? After further investigation you formulate this question: In this otherwise healthy 75-year-old woman with knee osteoarthritis can glucosamine/chondroitin improve symptoms and joint motility? In DARE, you find this meta-analysis: Richy F, Bruyere O, Ethgen O, et al. Structural and symptomatic efficacy of glucosamine and chondroitin in knee osteoarthritis. A comprehensive meta-analysis. *Arch Intern Med.* 2003;163:1514–22.

Read the article, and formulate a recommendation for the patient. Use the appropriate critical appraisal worksheet provided as a tool at the end of this appendix.

Critical Appraisal Worksheet: Case–Control (Harm) Trials

Checklist	Comments
Questions addressed by the study are:	
Is the study design suitable for the objective?	
Did the exposure precede outcome?	
Was the control group identical to the cases other than the exposure? ≻ Were confounders identified and accounted for in the analysis?	
Was exposure ascertained adequately? ≻ Are subjective or objective measurements used to ascertain outcome? ≻ Was assessment performed in the same manner for all groups?	

Adapted with permission from Centre for Evidence-Based Medicine: www.cebm.net (select "appraisal" under "doing EBM").

Critical Appraisal Worksheet: Cohort (Prognosis) Trials

Checklist	Comments
Questions addressed by the study are:	
Is this study the best design to answer the question?	
Is the study relevant to your information needs in terms of ≻ Population? ≻ Risk factors studies? ≻ Outcome reported?	
Was recruitment adequate? ≻ Was the cohort representative of the desired population?	
Was the exposure accurately measured? ≻ Are subjective or objective measurements used to ascertain exposure?	
Was the outcome accurately measured? ≻ Are subjective or objective measurements used to ascertain outcome? ≻ Has a reliable system been established for detecting all cases?	
Was follow-up sufficiently long? ≻ Did more than 80% of the subjects complete the trial? ≻ Was the follow-up sufficiently long to reveal the beneficial and adverse effects?	
Were confounders identified and accounted for? ≻ Was analysis performed to correct, control, or adjust for confounding factors?	

Adapted with permission from Centre for Evidence-Based Medicine: www.cebm.net (select "appraisal" under "doing EBM").

Critical Appraisal Worksheet: Randomized Controlled (Efficacy/Safety) Trials

Checklist	Comments
Is the study valid? Questions addressed by the study are: ➤ Is the study relevant to your information needs (remember PICO—patient, intervention, comparison, and outcome)? ➤ Is the study best answered by a controlled trial?	
Was the study randomized? ➤ Was the word *randomized* or a related word (e.g., *random, randomly*) used? ➤ Was a method used to balance the randomization from known confounders (e.g., block design, stratification)?	
Was the random allocation concealed? ➤ A randomization method is adequate if it allows each participant to have the same chance of receiving each drug and if the investigator could not predict which drug was next. ➤ How was random allocation generated?	
Was randomization successful? ➤ Were important prognostic determinants evenly distributed (i.e., were the groups comparable at baseline)? ➤ Were any baseline differences between the groups reported? ➤ Could differences at entry between the groups explain the differences in outcome?	
Was the study double-blinded? ➤ Was the word *double-blinded* used? ➤ Was neither the person accessing the outcome nor the patient able to identify the treatment? ➤ Was blinding successful? ➤ Did participants guess their allocation?	
Were the groups treated equally aside from the experimental drug therapy? ➤ Was any group more likely to receive co-intervention? ➤ Were subjects in both groups followed at the same time intervals?	
Was intention-to-treat analysis performed? ➤ Were all patients analyzed in the group to which they were randomized?	

Critical Appraisal Worksheet: Randomized Controlled (Efficacy/Safety) Trials (continued)

Was relatively complete follow-up achieved? ➤ Were the reasons for withdrawals given? ➤ Were more than 80% of the randomized subjects completed?	
Was sample size large enough? ➤ Is there a description of the author's power calculation?	

Adapted with permission from Centre for Evidence-Based Medicine: www.cebm.net (select "appraisal" under "doing EBM").

Critical Appraisal Worksheet: Systematic Reviews of Randomized Controlled Trials

Checklist	Comments
Is the review valid? Questions addressed by the review are: ➤ Is the review relevant to your information needs (remember PICO—patient, intervention, comparison, and outcome)? ➤ Does the review address a focused question that is likely to be answered by a systematic review?	
Were all relevant trials found? ➤ Which databases were searched? ➤ Was the search strategy comprehensive? ➤ Was pearling used? ➤ Were experts consulted?	
Were the criteria used to include trials appropriate? ➤ Was the appropriate trial design selected? ➤ Was the appropriate PICO selected?	
Was the selection of primary studies free of bias? ➤ Is the methodology reproducible? ➤ Was more than one reviewer applying inclusion criteria to prevent selection bias?	
Was the validity/quality of the included individual trials assessed? ➤ Was a quality scale/scoring system used?	
Were the results similar from trial to trial? ➤ Are the results graphically displayed so that you can visually ascertain whether results were fairly similar? ➤ Are the results homogeneous or heterogeneous?	

Adapted with permission from Centre for Evidence-Based Medicine: www.cebm.net (select "appraisal" under "doing EBM").

APPENDIX 3–C
ADDITIONAL SUGGESTED READING ON CRITICAL APPRAISAL SKILLS

The Public Health Resource Unit's Web site (http://www.phru.nhs.uk/casp/casp.htm) provides useful and easy checklists. You can select the article to be critically appraised, decide the type of study, and then download the relevant checklist. By answering the questions in the checklist, you will reach a conclusion about the usefulness of the article. In addition, there are non-virtual workshops to which you may subscribe, but these may lack the benefit of convenience offered by online learning.

The CATbank. At the Centre for Evidence-Based Medicine in Oxford (http://www.cebm.net/cats.asp), the Critically Appraised Topics Program, "CAT", is a simple software program that helps clinicians to summarize the evidence. The program can be used to save any critical appraisal you have done on a previous occasion.

The Critical Appraisal Skill Programme offers several tools on their Web site to learn more about critical appraisal:
http://www.pdptoolkit.co.uk/Files/ebm/indexes/guide%20to%20ebm.htm.

The BMJ Publishing Group offers a How to Read a Paper series in both print and online issues of the *BMJ* (http://bmj.bmjjournals.com/collections/read.dtl):

- Papers that report drug trials. *BMJ.* 1997;315:480–3; http://www.bmj.com/cgi/content/full/315/7106/480
- Papers that tell you what things cost (economic analyses). *BMJ.* 1997;315:596–9; http://www.bmj.com/cgi/content/full/315/7108/596
- Papers that summarise other papers (systematic reviews and meta-analyses). *BMJ.* 1997;315:672–5; http://www.bmj.com/cgi/content/full/315/7109/672
- Papers that go beyond numbers (qualitative research). *BMJ.* 1997;315:740–3; http://www.bmj.com/cgi/content/full/315/7110/740

This group also offers a *BMJ* collection of articles relevant to the critical appraisal of systematic reviews: http://bmj.bmjjournals.com/collections/ma.htm.

The Centre for Health Evidence provides a series of articles based on the series Users' Guides to Evidence-Based Medicine, originally published in *JAMA*:

- Therapy and prevention: http://www.cche.net/principles/content_therapy.asp
- Harm: http://www.cche.net/principles/content_harm.asp
- Overview articles: http://www.cche.net/principles/content_overview.asp
- Clinical decision analyses: http://www.cche.net/principles/content_d_analysis.asp
- Clinical practice guidelines: http://www.cche.net/principles/content_p_guideline.asp
- Clinical utilization reviews: http://www.cche.net/principles/content_u_review.asp
- Outcomes of health service research:
  http://www.cche.net/principles/content_v_outcome.asp
- Quality of life measures: http://www.cche.net/principles/content_qol.asp
- Economic analyses: http://www.cche.net/principles/content_e_analysis.asp
- Grading health care recommendations:
  http://www.cche.net/principles/content_grading.asp
- Applicability of clinical trials results:
  http://www.cche.net/principles/content_results.asp

Additional Tutorials with Worked Examples

➤ Written by Alan O'Rourke, this University of Sheffield tutorial provides the basic critical appraisal skills for primary resources but also introduces how to evaluate a Web site: http://www.shef.ac.uk/scharr/ir/units/critapp/index.htm.

➤ Evaluating the Studies You Find workshop, produced by the SUNY Downstate Medical Center, is another valuable resource: http://servers.medlib.hscbklyn.edu/ebm/5toc.htm.

4

DEMYSTIFYING STATISTICS

Gilbert Ramirez

*T*HIS IS THE AGE OF EVIDENCE-BASED PRACTICE. Conceptualization of this chapter began with an Internet search using the phrase "evidence-based." Not surprisingly, the search resulted in 6,300,000 hits. A modest but reasonable collection of evidence-based texts covers a wide array of disciplines including medicine, herbal medicine, public health, health promotion, health economics, and health policy. At a recent national conference, several evidence-based texts in other disciplines such as cardiology, dentistry, and nursing were displayed. A brochure for the 2004 annual conference of the American Association of University Programs in Health Administration announced the theme "Evidence-Based Health Services Management." Furthermore, countless texts and papers on evidence-based methodologies (including systematic reviews and meta-analysis) are available, and evidence-based professional collaborations such as the Cochrane (http://www.cochrane.org) and the Campbell Collaborations (http://www.campbellcollaboration.org) are undergoing great growth.

So much has been written under the evidence-based mantra, one wonders what could a statistician contribute that would be of any value beyond what is already available in the countless texts and papers, especially in the area of statistics. Most clinicians often take only one statistics course required as part of professional training. One does not have to be a statistician to use statistics; one simply needs to be able to correctly interpret statistical results. That skill is easily learned. Statistics is about probability, and using statistics is about minimizing the probability of making a poor decision. If one were to ask, "Why statistics?" the answer would be "to make the best decision possible with the available evidence."

In the study of statistics, we tend to focus on measures such as the mean (or average), the risk (or probability of an outcome occurring), or the relative risk (the risk in one group divided by the risk in a comparison group), and so on. But we often forget that these measures are a function of the degree of differences among those studied, and that the degree of differences also contributes to the degree of uncertainty for which the findings can be used in making decisions.

This chapter will attempt to demystify statistics by examining the issue of "differences" as it contributes to four elements: variability, magnitude of effect, relationships between constructs (or variables), and strength of the evidence. Appendix 4–A provides a glossary of the terms often encountered in discussions of these and other statistical elements.

Examination of variability will include (1) exploration of how "differences" contribute to the various measures of central tendency, or "points of reference"; (2) exploration of how these differences contribute to measures of dispersion, or "points of departure"; and (3) examination of how statistical significance ("a roll of the dice") differs from clinical or substantive significance ("my dad is bigger than your dad").

How the contribution of differences to statistics is measured (through variability) and evaluated (by using magnitudes of effect) will be discussed. Then, an examination of the ways variables can be described with respect to each other or, in other words, "how they are related" will be presented. This examination will include relationships from the simplest bivariate situation to the more complex multivariate scenario. Finally, the factors that contribute to the strength of evidence, such as differences between study designs and the use of different statistical methods, will be discussed.

Examining Variability

Variability is a relative concept—for variability to exist, a sense of departure from some reference point must be present. Introductory statistics text typically begins with a discussion of measures of central tendency (mean, median, and mode) followed by measures of dispersion (e.g., variance, standard deviation, and standard error of the mean). Variability may be described from a directional perspective (e.g., a uniform or nonuniform increase or decrease from a stated point of reference). In pharmacotherapy, directional departures from an established reference, such as "improvement in patient outcome," are usually of more interest.

Measures of Central Tendency: "Points of Reference"

The three most commonly used (and most often described in statistical texts) measures of central tendency are the mean, median, and mode. The mean (or simply the "average" as described in elementary school) is the most often used—and misused—statistic. Misuse of the mean (instead of, for example, the median) can invalidate a claim of statistical significance. "Consumers of statistics" commonly focus their reading of the evidence on whether a finding is (or is not) statistically significant, and rarely question whether the data that went into the determination of statistical significance were appropriate, ignoring the reality that findings based on invalid methods can be statistically significant too.

The mean, or simple average, is used for continuous data that are normally (or reasonably) distributed (i.e., have a bell-shape appearance when the values are plotted along the X-axis and the frequency of each value is plotted along the Y-axis of a graph). When the data are not continuous but are ordinal, the appropriate measure of central tendency to use is the median. Data can be continuous but skewed (i.e., distribution is "almost normal," but instead of a perfectly shaped bell, the data are either skewed negatively [left-hand side of bell is elongated] or skewed positively). In this case the data must either be transformed before parametric statistical tests can be performed so that their distribution is normal (the mean would then be an appropriate measure of central tendency) or the median must be used. To transform data, one typically multiplies the data by some factor (a logarithm for example) so that the transformed data take on the characteristic bell-shaped curve. The mode is used to describe nonordinal, categorical variables such as race/ethnicity, socioeconomic status, or administration route of a medication (e.g., orally, intravenously, subcutaneously).

Unfortunately, reports of research findings usually do not provide sufficient information about the data to allow determination of whether the appropriate measure of central tendency was used. Many details of the study have to be left out because of limits placed on the submitting authors by journal editors. Someone who is familiar with the literature in a certain field may also be familiar with other articles in which the underlying distribution of similar data has been reported. These alternative articles can be used to make judgments about the use and misuse of specific statistical measures. The peer-review process of selected journals is also a safeguard, but certainly not a guarantee that appropriate statistical measures have been used in a particular study. However, the evidence can be examined to see if the measure(s) of dispersion are appropriate for the reported measure(s) of central tendency.

Measures of Dispersion: Points of Departure

Once the correct measure of central tendency has been chosen, the next question is matching that with an appropriate measure of dispersion of the data. When means have been selected to measure and report central tendency, the appropriate measure of dispersion is the standard deviation (SD), which is the square root of the variance. The appropriate measure of dispersion when the median has been reported is the interquartile range. When central tendency has been reported as modes, the only way to describe departure is to report the percentage (or proportion, or frequency) of observations in the categories other than the modal category.

Often, consumers of statistics and sometimes even researchers will confuse the SD statistic with the standard error (SE), and this mistake can be important. The SD is a measure of variability within a population, but the standard error is a measure of the uncertainty of the sample mean as a true estimate of the population mean. For example, if a study (sample size = 25) reports an average cholesterol reduction of 25 mg/dL with an SD of 5 mg/dL, 95% of the population is expected to fall within ± 2 SDs of the mean. It would be unusual (less than 5% of the time) to observe a reduction of less than 15 mg/dL or greater than 35 mg/dL.

The SE (or standard error of the mean [SEM]) is calculated as the SD divided by the square root of the sample size:

$$SEM = SD\!\!\Big/\!\!\sqrt{n}$$

For the cholesterol reduction example above, the SEM would be equal to 5 divided by the square root of 25, for an SEM value of 1.0; the SEM is then used to calculate a confidence interval (CI; a 95% CI is used in this example) and used to calculate a t statistic to test the hypothesis that the reduction differs from 0. The 95% CI for this example is calculated as follows:

$$95\%\,CI = \bar{X} \pm 2.06(SEM)$$

$$95\%\,CI = \bar{X} \pm 2.06\left(SD\!\!\Big/\!\!\sqrt{n}\right)$$

$$95\%\,CI = 25 \pm 2.06\left(5\!\!\Big/\!\!\sqrt{25}\right)$$

$$95\%\,CI = 25 \pm 2.06$$

$$95\%\,CI = 22.93 \text{ to } 27.06$$

If the calculation were based on a population rather than a sample, the number would be 1.96 (SDs). Because sample data with a sample size of 25 are being used, the number is 2.06

(obtained from a *t* statistics table, and based on a sample size of 25 and an alpha level of .05). The 95% CI of 22.93 mg/dL to 27.06 mg/dL differs remarkably from the range provided by the mean ± 2 SDs (15–35 mg/dL). The SEM, as stated previously, is a measure of the uncertainty of the sample mean as a true estimate of the population mean. In this example, the data suggest a 95% chance that the true population average is between 22.93 and 27.06 mg/dL, but says nothing about the range of "normal values" for the population as provided by the calculation using the SD. To interpret the same data for a range of "normal values" for a population, one should examine the prediction interval:

$$95\% \, PI = \bar{X} \pm 2.06 \left(SD \times \sqrt{1 + \frac{1}{n}} \right)$$

$$95\% \, PI = 25 \pm 2.06(5 \times 1.02)$$

$$95\% \, PI = 25 \pm 10.52$$

$$95\% \, PI = 14.48 \text{ to } 35.52$$

The 95% CI is the range of values that, when asked by a patient, "What results can I expect?" the practitioner can respond, "The average patient will have a cholesterol reduction somewhere between 22.9 to 27.1 mg/dL." Another answer might be "95% of patients will have a cholesterol reduction somewhere between 14.5 to 35.5 mg/dL, and it just depends where you are as an individual patient."

Statistics, the realm of researchers, are about "average patients"; practitioners work with all patients, and few are at the average. A good rule of thumb for estimating the prediction interval (rather than calculating the precise values when the researcher fails to report the prediction interval) is to subtract 2 SDs from the lower limit of the 95% CI and to add 2 SDs to the upper limit of the 95% CI. In this example, the rule of thumb would provide a range of values of (23 – 10) to (27 + 10) or 13 to 37 mg/dL (Figure 4–1).

It is useful to note that narrow CIs provide a more precise estimate of the population mean. An additional point about SDs and SEs: Researchers will sometimes report the SEM instead of the SD because the SEM is always smaller than the SD and, therefore, reporting the SEM makes their results appear more precise. There is no evidence to suggest that this substitution is intentional (to make their data look better), but it is useful to know the difference between these two measures when reviewing results.

While statistical software now typically prevents this type of error, researchers will sometimes substitute the SD for the SEM when conducting a statistical test (such as the *t* test). The denominator of the *t* test (or any statistical test) is the SEM. If the researcher uses instead the larger SD, the resulting value of the *t* statistic will be smaller than if it had been correctly calculated. The rule for determining when a research finding is statistically significant is as follows: If the value of the test statistic (e.g., *t* statistic) is greater than the value from a set of values in the *t* distribution table, the finding is statistically significant. (Another issue is whether the correct value from the table has been chosen, which will be addressed later.) If SD is used instead of SEM when calculating the *t* statistic, the result will be smaller than it should and may be the determining factor for a finding to be nonsignificant when, in fact, it is significant. Similarly, a CI is determined on the basis of the SEM. When CI is calculated using SD instead, the result is a wider CI, which is a more "conservative" interpretation of the results (and the wider the CI, the less likely a finding will be found to be statistically significant). Being "more

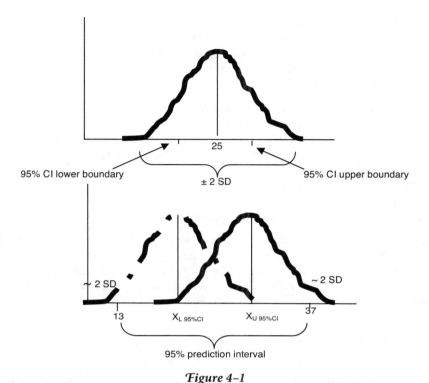

Figure 4-1
CI (around a mean) and prediction interval (around the upper and lower limits of the CI).

conservative" is a "better mistake" than the opposite, but if the mistake is made, an effective therapy may appear not to be effective.

Sometimes researchers will plot their results using SEM instead of SD. When this is done, the study appears to be more "precise" because the smaller SEM value gives the appearance of less variability (synonymous with more precision), and the report therefore would be a candidate for that classic book *How to Lie with Statistics*. The bottom line is that we need to know, as journal readers and users of the literature, when it is appropriate to use SEM and when to use SD.

Magnitudes of Effect

Magnitude of effect, as represented by the effect size statistic, is a concept central to meta-analysis and evidence-based practice. The value of a statistical test (such as the *t* statistic), sample size, and effect size are all distinctly and directly related. As sample size increases, so does the value of the statistical test, which increases the likelihood of a statistically significant finding (even when the clinical importance of the finding is minimal). As effect size increases, so does the value of the statistical test.

The value of the statistical test is indirectly related to the probability that an observed event occurred by chance alone: the larger the value of the statistical test, the lower the probability (*P* value) of chance as an explanation for the observed finding. Another way of saying this is that a statistically significant finding is not likely the result of chance.

Consumers of statistics have been conditioned to focus more on statistical significance and less on clinical significance (substantive or practical significance, or clinical relevance or importance). Statistical significance is a function of the value of the statistical test, while clinical significance is a function of the effect size alone. The mathematical relationships among statistical significance, sample size, and effect size suggest the following questions for examination of evidence:

> ➤ When the result is statistically significant,
>   —Is the effect size of substantive or clinical importance?
>   —Is the sample size simply large—that is, has a very small difference reached statistical significance simply because so many patients or observations are included in the data set?
> ➤ When the result is not statistically significant,
>   —Is the effect size of substantive or clinical importance?
>   —Is perhaps the sample size simply too small?

When the sample size is too small, the study is described as having too little power to detect the effect. Unfortunately, many of these situations go unnoticed because studies tend not to be published when the results are not statistically significant. In "published" studies, the reader must consider how clinically relevant the observed outcome is, even if it very likely represents a real difference between treatments and not the result of chance alone.

Statistical Significance: "A Role of the Dice"

The significance of a statistical test is the probability that an observed effect could occur by chance alone. The probability of an observed effect occurring by chance alone is addressed at two points in a study: at the beginning when designing the study and considering the level of confidence/significance desired (α, or alpha level), and at the end when analyzing the data (P value, or probability value).

Most historians agree that the interest and need for statistical methods evolved from the interest in probability and, in particular, the probabilities associated with games of chance. Whether throwing dice or playing a round of poker, the knowledge of the probability of events (combinations of numbers or cards) is the only honest way (other than pure luck) to consistently make good decisions (as the song says, "You have to know when to hold them, know when to fold them"). In science, studies are commonly designed at an alpha level of .05, which can be interpreted as being willing to accept a 5% (or less) chance of being wrong (i.e., an observed result is not true)—a type I error. Two questions are important to address with respect to alpha levels of 5% (or any value): Why 5%? What does 5% mean in terms of a single study?

There is no logical rationale for a 5% alpha level other than this value is used most often. Statistical texts abound with examples of 5% alphas and 95% CIs. Some investigators say the 5% alpha level is based on the well-known "monkey see, monkey do" principle.

When is an observed event statistically significant? It is statistically significant (not likely to be explained by chance alone) when the P value (a function of the data) is less than the alpha level (set by the investigator). For a given set of data (and a given statistical test), the P value is fixed; therefore, whether the results are statistically significant depends entirely on what alpha level has been chosen (hopefully before examining the data) by the investigator. Investigators will sometimes report a result as "almost statistically significant" or state that "a statistical trend was present." For example, when the P value of .06 is obtained and the investigator had chosen an alpha level of .05, the temptation is great to point to a small sample size or other factor in the statistical calculations. There is, however, no such thing as "almost significant"—it either is or it is not. The important consideration is whether the investigator chose an alpha level appropriate for the research question.

The level of alpha that is appropriate to the question being asked depends on the implications of making a wrong decision. Statistical texts refer to this event as the type I error, or the error committed in rejecting a false null hypothesis when, in fact, the hypothesis is true. Decisions to act (change course of action) are made when the null hypothesis is rejected. For example, in a new pharmaceutical therapy, the null hypothesis would state something along the line: "The new therapy is as effective or less effective than the standard therapy." Naturally, the manufacturer hopes that the drug is actually more effective so that it can proceed with marketing the drug Assuming that the data suggest the new drug appears more effective than the standard therapy, when the clinician asks, "How likely is this observation due to chance alone?" the answer is "less than 5%" (P value < .05). On the basis of the P value being less than our accepted alpha level of .05, the clinician would reject the null hypothesis and accept the alternative hypothesis that the new drug is indeed more effective (with less than a 5% chance of this conclusion being wrong). If the "truth" is that the new drug is more effective, then the conclusion is good, and a decision to act (change to the new drug) would be a good decision. If the truth is that the standard therapy is actually more effective, then the rejection of the null hypothesis and acceptance of the alternative hypothesis would be an incorrect conclusion, and any decision to act would be a bad decision. Because for any set of data there is only one P value and, therefore, statistical conclusions (to reject or not to reject) are based on the study's alpha level, at what level should alpha be set?

The primary criterion for setting alpha from a decision-making perspective is the severity of the potential implication of a bad decision (there are other statistical criteria, but that is beyond the scope of this chapter). The greater the severity, the more we want to be sure that we do not make a bad decision; therefore, using lower alpha levels should be considered. For example, if an alpha level of .05 is used as a starting point, how severe is the implication of making a bad decision when the decision to be made is life-and-death (e.g., whether to have open heart surgery)? While the severity is difficult to quantify exactly, most clinicians would probably want to minimize the probability of a bad decision to something less than 5%, perhaps 1%. In contrast, what alpha level is appropriate for a decision that is not life-and-death? For example, if the decision is whether to use a new health promotion pamphlet when there is still a good supply of the old pamphlet in storage (represents costs), an alpha level of 5% seems appropriate or at least more appropriate than for the open heart surgery example. Taking it a step further, what if the decision to be made is about what color to paint classroom walls on the basis of the hypothesis that color is related to learning. In this scenario, an alpha greater than 5% might be okay. Why would one even consider alpha levels greater than 5%? The answer is a smaller alpha level requires a larger sample size, which in turn increases the cost of the study. It is important to note that .05 is an accepted industry standard, and setting alpha higher than .05 could be subject to criticism by many in the scientific community.

What does 5% mean in terms of a single study? When an alpha or significance level of 5% is chosen as the criterion, this is a statement that the researcher is willing to "live" with the possibility of making a type I error 5% of the time. Accepting an error rate of 5% is the complement of being 95% confident. A 95% CI is a statement that "in 95 of 100 similar studies, the true population parameter value would be included in the range of possible values represented by the study's 95% CI." Statistics are estimates of the population parameter, and much of statistics is about how good the statistic is at estimating the population parameter. A type I error can occur at any time: the 50th time a study is conducted, the 96th time a study is conducted, and even the first time a study is conducted.

Substantive Significance: "My dad is bigger than your dad."

〜
Scenario
〜

A friend read in her magazine that taking garlic could decrease her cholesterol levels. She asked your opinion. You pulled a meta-analysis recently published in Archives of Internal Medicine *addressing the effect of garlic on cardiovascular risk factors. The authors reported that garlic decreased total cholesterol by 12 mg/dL (95% CI, –23.6 to –0.5 mg/dL) with a corresponding effect size of –0.3 (95% CI, –0.6 to –0.01), both significant decreases from a statistical standpoint.*

As discussed earlier, substantive (or clinical, or practical) significance indicates a measured change in the outcome of interest of sufficient magnitude on which to base a decision for therapeutic change. The "change" is also referred to as the "effect size" and may be measured in the original units of the outcome of interest, or in a unitless statistic (these will be described in more detail later in the chapter in the section Relationships) such as a standardized mean difference, odds ratio/relative risk, difference in relative frequency, or correlation coefficient. Table 4–1 provides a scale for interpreting "how substantive" an effect size is.

When examining evidence from a single study, it is important to consider both statistical and substantive significance. Is the magnitude of effect of sufficient size to justify a therapeutic change? If it is, how likely is the observed effect due to chance alone—is the finding statistically significant? Or could it simply be that this study is in the "5% of studies" that do not include the true population effect size? What if the effect is substantively but not statistically significant? Did the study have a large enough sample size (power) to detect the observed effect? The latter issue of power analysis, unfortunately, is beyond the scope of this chapter, but readers are encouraged to explore this important issue in greater depth with other readings or a statistician.

Table 4–1 Substantivity of Effect Size

Effect Size	Trivial	Small	Moderate	Large	Very Large	Nearly Perfect	Perfect
Standardized mean difference	0	0.2	0.6	1.2	2.0	4.0	Infinite
OR	1.0	1.5	3.5	9.0	32	360	Infinite
RR	1.0	1.2	1.9	3.0	5.7	19	Infinite
Relative frequency difference	0	10	30	50	70	90	100
r	0	0.1	0.3	0.5	0.7	0.9	1

OR = Odds ratio; RR = relative risk; r = correlation coefficient.

Source: Adapted with permission from Sportscience Web site. A new view of statistics. Available at: http://www.sportsci.org/resource/stats/effectmag.html. Accessed October 17, 2006. Copyright 2006 Will G. Hopkins.

Relationships

Rarely is a single construct or variable of interest. The answer to the question "what is the prevalence of diabetes?" has little value by itself. The types of questions that interest us in health care are relational ones such as:

➤ What is the difference in the prevalence of diabetes in population A and population B?
➤ Is population A at greater risk for developing diabetes than population B?
➤ Has the incidence of diabetes in population A decreased during the past 5 years?
➤ Is there an improvement in quality of life among patients with diabetes undergoing treatment with therapy X versus treatment with therapy Y?

These are questions about the relationship between disease prevalence and membership in a particular population; between the risk of developing diabetes and population membership; and between the incidence of disease and time, quality of life, and type of therapy, respectively. Statistical measures for describing bivariate relationships such as these are typically one of the following: measures of covariation, measures of differences, or relative measures.

Measures of Covariation

Statistics of covariation include the Pearson and the Spearman correlation coefficients. Correlation coefficients measure the degree to which two variables covary, that is, the degree to which one variable changes when the other changes. The possible values for correlation coefficients range from –1 to +1, with 0 representing the "null value" or no relationship between the two variables. When both variables change in the same direction (e.g., as one becomes increasingly positive or negative, so does the other), the relationship is described as "positive correlation," and the correlation coefficient is $0 < r \leq +1$. When the two variables change in different directions (one positive, the other negative; or vice versa), the relationship is described as a "negative correlation," and the correlation coefficient is $-1 \leq r < 0$. When a change in one variable occurs with no change in the other variable, the relationship is described as "no correlation," and the correlation coefficient is $r = 0$. But $r = 0$ can also occur when the relationship is nonlinear. For this reason, the data should be plotted before calculation of a correlation coefficient to make sure the relationship appears linear, not curvilinear.

The Pearson correlation coefficient is used when both variables have been measured on a continuous scale, and the Spearman correlation coefficient when one or both variables have been measured on an ordinal scale. When reviewing evidence that reports correlation coefficients, the direction of the relationship (positive or negative) as well as the magnitude (distance from 0) should be considered. When the magnitude of the relationship appears substantive (Table 4–1), the probability that this effect could have occurred by chance alone (is it statistically significant?) should be considered. When assessing statistical significance, the CI should be considered: If the coefficient is statistically significant, the CI will *not* include the null value 0; both limits will be either positive or negative. Other considerations include the following: How significant is the relationship? How small is the *P* value? Is it .049 or .005? How close is the lower CI (or upper CI, when the correlation is negative) to the null value 0?

Related to the correlation coefficient (r) is the coefficient of determination (r^2). The correlation coefficient measures the degree of association between two variables and ranges from 0, or no association, to +1. The coefficient of determination measures the proportion of variability explained in one variable (such as the dependent variable in a regression analysis) by another variable (the independent variable in the regression analysis). The coefficient of determination is also a good measure of "how well" the regression equation (sometimes called the regression model) explains variation observed in the dependent variable (the model can have one or more independent variables). The coefficient of determination ranges from 0 to +1; because it is the squared value of r, it cannot be a negative value. A value of 0 suggests that the model does not explain any of the variation, while a value of 1 suggests that the model explains all of the variation. Coefficients of determination are always smaller in magnitude than the correlation coefficient: An *r* of .5 might appear impressive, but its corresponding r^2 value is only .25 (which also means 25% of the variability in the values of Y is explained by the values of X).

Measures of Difference

Statistics that measure differences include the difference between means (independent samples or paired), the difference between rates and proportions (risk difference/absolute risk), and the standardized mean difference (*z* scores). Common to each of these "difference" statistics is the null value 0; therefore, a simple check of the results from a reviewer's perspective is "does the CI exclude 0 when the investigator has reported a statistically significant finding?" If 0 is included within the limits of the interval, the result *cannot* be statistically significant at the specified CI level—something is wrong!

Reporting of the *z* score has increased as interest in and support for meta-analysis have grown. Simply stated, the standardized mean difference is the difference between two means, divided by a SD (typically the pooled SD). What results, the *z* score, is a unitless statistic, meaning that, if the original means were reported as milligram per deciliter (mg/dL) units, when their difference is divided by the SD (also reported in milligram per deciliter units), the units cancel out. The resulting statistic, therefore, has no unit other than what can be described as a "standard deviation unit." This approach is useful in many statistical situations, but has relatively little value to the practitioner. The rules for statistical significance are the same (does the CI include 0?), but the interpretation and generalization of a *z* score for use in practice (whatever the practice) leaves a lot to be desired. Hopefully, the investigator has provided some "translation" of the standardized mean differences observed, but if not, there is a simple procedure one can use to "translate" the *z* scores. The following equation is the first step:

$$z_{\text{score}} = \frac{\bar{X}_1 - \bar{X}_2}{SD_{\text{pooled}}}$$

After using "basic algebraic manipulation" and providing a value for the question "what is the typical SD for this population?" the following equation is obtained:

$$\bar{X}_1 - \bar{X}_2 = (z_{\text{score}})(SD_{\text{pooled}})$$

This simple approach provides a way to convert or translate *z* scores into more meaningful statistics: the difference between means as expressed in the original unit (e.g., milligram per deciliter as used in the earlier example). Most of us have a sense of what the typical SD is in our particular areas of interest, but if not, one can review other similar studies and obtain an estimate through averaging. Also, one could use a range of possible SD values and then produce a range of possible mean differences. The same technique can be used to convert CIs for standardized mean differences into the CIs with the original units. For example, in Figure 4–2 the data represent studies from a meta-analysis of the relationship between garlic and cholesterol levels. The original studies had reported cholesterol change in milligram per deciliter units, and the researchers on this project chose to convert these units to effect size units before integrating (horizontal axis at top of graph). Then, effect size units (*z* scores) were "translated" into clinically meaningful units by converting the top axis effect size values to milligram per

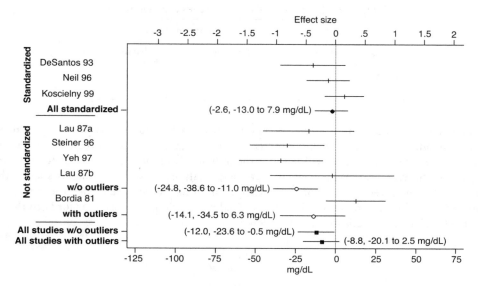

Figure 4–2

Converting effect sizes to mean differences using data from a meta-analysis of studies of the effect of garlic on serum cholesterol studies. (Agency for Healthcare Quality and Research. Garlic: effects on cardiovascular risks and disease, protective effects against cancer, and clinical adverse effects. Available at: http://www.ahrq.gov/clinic/tp/garlictp.htm. Accessed November 1, 2006.)

deciliter units (bottom horizontal axis) by multiplying the mean and lower/upper CIs (effect sizes) by the value 40.8 mg/dL. The conversion factor of 40.8 was taken from the average of the SD values from all of the studies included in the meta-analysis. Readers were cautioned, however, that the actual values for milligram per deciliter would depend on the value used to convert the effect sizes; if one thought the SD should be higher, then the higher value could easily be substituted by using the same process described above.

Relative to the discussion on substantive significance and comparison of the standardized mean difference effect size scale on the upper X-axis, a small effect is 0.2, moderate is 0.6, and large is 1.2; the overall effect of garlic in this example would appear to be small to moderate.

Relative Relationships

A very useful measure for comparison is one that describes the relative magnitudes between two univariate statistics. The most common measures are the relative risk (RR), or risk ratio, and the odds ratio (OR). The null value (no difference between groups) for both relative statistics is 1; therefore, the CIs should exclude 1 when the finding is reported as statistically significant. The statistic is a ratio between two numbers such as two incidence rates. A value greater than 1 indicates the group represented by the rate in the numerator is more likely to have the outcome of interest than the group represented by the rate in the denominator. Conversely, a value less than 1 indicates the group represented by the numerator is less likely to have the outcome.

Table 4-2   2 × 2 Factorial for Relative Risk and Odds Ratio

Risk Factor?	Outcome of Interest?	
	Present	Absent
Yes	a	b
No	c	d

The RR and OR are similar measures, and under certain conditions (when the prevalence of the outcome of interest is low), the OR is a good estimate of the RR, which is the measure of choice for prospective studies. The OR is the only measure that can be calculated with retrospective study designs. When reviewing a meta-analysis, most methodologists agree that the OR is the preferred measure of effect when combining studies, even when the studies are prospective and RRs were reported in the original publication. The formulas for both the RR and the OR, based on Table 4–2, are as follows:

$$RR = \frac{a / (a+b)}{c / (c+d)}$$

$$OR = \frac{ad}{bc}$$

Hazard Ratio

The hazard ratio (HR) is similar to the RR; the terms are sometimes used interchangeably. The true *hazard ratio*, however, can be described as a longitudinal extension of the RR as described earlier. When data are examined from a survival perspective, using time-to-event measures (the length of time during which no event was observed), individual subjects contribute the additional information of event-free time. The appropriate way to summarize time-to-event data when comparing two groups is the HR. This measure is interpreted in a similar way to the RR, and specifically as how much more (or less) likely an individual in one group is to suffer an event at a particular point in time compared with an individual in a comparison group.

Multivariate Relationships

Health care studies, and life in general, are far more complex than the two-variable perspectives presented above. Multivariate analyses afford a researcher the opportunity to explore relationships between multiple variables at the same time. Most of these examinations are functions and/or extensions of the multiple regression model. Variations to this model are based on the nature of the dependent variable (is it continuous, categorical, or dichotomous?) and the nature of the independent variables (are they linear or nonlinear?). Some other considerations include the following: How are missing data handled? Are the results based on a full model or a reduced model generated by a stepwise procedure? If stepwise, was it a forward, backward, or all-way stepwise procedure? The issues related to multivariate models are many and beyond the scope of this chapter; readers are encouraged to seek out other texts and/or a good statistician.

∽
Scenario
∽

A total of 118 patients with mild-to-moderate essential hypertension were randomized to treatment with 10 mg/day of amlodipine (Norvasc—Pfizer Inc.), 20 mg/day of quinapril (Accupril—Pfizer Inc.), or 100 mg/day of losartan (Cozaar—Merck & Co., Inc.). Analysis of differences in time was performed by means of multiple analyses of variance (ANOVAs) with repeated measurements. In the presence of significant effects, post hoc analysis (Scheffé test) was carried out.

It is useful, however, to discuss in some detail the use of ANOVA. Basically, when the dependent variable is continuous and the independent variable is categorical, ANOVA is the preferred method to describe the relationship between the two variables. ANOVA is typically used when the categorical variable is based on three or more groupings. Although ANOVA could be used when the categorical variable is based on only two groupings, this situation is usually examined by using the independent or paired *t* test.

The error most often made when using ANOVA is the interpretation of a statistically significant finding. The null hypothesis for ANOVA is that the means of all groups are equal. When the null hypothesis is rejected (indicating statistical significance), the correct interpretation of the alternative hypothesis is that *at least two* of the group means differ, not that *all* of the group means differ. When the null hypothesis has been rejected, the investigator is limited to knowing not only that *at least two* of the group means differ, but also to *not* knowing *which* group means differ. To determine the latter, the investigator must use a multiple comparison test, of which there are several to choose from (e.g., Bonferroni, Tukey Honestly Significant Difference [HSD], Scheffé, Newman–Keuls, and Dunnet procedures).

When the investigator plans multiple comparisons a priori (before the data are collected), then the Bonferroni test is appropriate. For example, a study may include four groups, one of which is a control group. The investigator is not interested in all possible comparisons, but only three: each of the three treatment groups compared with the control group. The three comparisons would be used to determine the value of the Bonferroni *t* statistic for this planned analysis. If the investigator were also interested in the comparison between two of the three treatment groups, there would be four comparisons, and the Bonferroni statistic would have a different value. Each comparison is then between two groups, and the Bonferroni statistic, which is essentially a *t* statistic, can be interpreted similarly. The key issues are the number of comparisons and that the comparisons are planned a priori. It was noted previously that there are statistical considerations for criteria for alpha levels. A multiple comparison procedure in effect reduces the study's alpha level for each of the multiple comparisons. For example, if the overall study alpha level is designed at .05, the multiple comparison procedure will use a lower alpha (e.g., .025, .01) for each of the subsequent comparisons. For the Bonferroni procedure, the alpha is adjusted by a factor depending on the number of comparisons being made. If there are three groups (A, B, and C) and group A is being compared with group B, group A with group B, and group B with group C (three comparisons), an overall study alpha of .05 would be adjusted to .05/3, or .017 for each of the three tests. The rationale for this adjustment is that, on the basis of chance alone, when multiple comparisons are being conducted, the likelihood of one comparison being significant increases. The procedure minimizes this likelihood by setting a lower alpha level, making it more difficult for an observed difference to be significant. This scenario (a significant finding by chance alone when many comparisons are being conducted) is referred to as the "fishing expedition" problem.

When multiple comparisons are considered after the data have been collected and analyzed, the investigator must use a post hoc comparison test instead of an a priori test (e.g., Bonferroni). Four of the multiple comparison tests listed above are appropriate in this instance. The Tukey HSD is used for only pair-wise comparisons, while the Scheffé test can be used for all possible comparisons (see previous scenario for an appropriate use of a post hoc test). The Scheffé value is larger than the Tukey HSD (for determining a statistically significant difference) and is therefore more conservative. The Newman–Keuls test uses a stepwise procedure and can only be used for pair-wise comparisons. The Dunnet procedure is used only in situations such as that described above for a planned comparison in which multiple treatment groups are compared with a single control group. A more detailed discussion of the advantages and disadvantages of each of these and other post hoc comparison tests is beyond the scope of this chapter, and readers are encouraged again to consult other statistical texts and/or a statistician. A useful rule of thumb when the researcher has not adjusted for multiple comparisons is to simply divide the overall study alpha by the number of comparisons (e.g., .05/3 = .017) and then compare the P value of each comparison made. In this example, if the P value is less than .017 (instead of less than .05), the comparison is statistically significant.

Strength of the Evidence

Two factors determine the strength of the evidence. The first is the design of the study: To what degree does the design minimize threats to validity? The second is the method used to analyze the data: To what degree are the statistical methods appropriate to the data collected? Readers are referred to Chapter 3 for a general discussion of study designs.

Scenario

A colleague is reviewing the POSITIVE trial for the next journal club. He asks you to explain the statistics behind this noninferiority trial. The primary end point occurred in 14% of patients assigned to the new drug and 14.5% of patients assigned to the gold standard (OR, 0.96; 95% CI, 0.86–1.06). The new drug was not superior to the gold standard, but was noninferior. In the Methods section, the authors report setting the upper boundary for the noninferiority claim at less than 1.1.

A study design that has utility in pharmacotherapy is the noninferiority trial. This adaptation of the randomized control trial is one in which a new therapy is compared with a standard active therapy instead of a placebo or untreated control group. The premise of the noninferiority trial is that for the new therapy to be "worthy," it needs to be only "as good" as the active control with respect to appropriate response outcomes. It is somewhat analogous to the premise of an "equivalence trial" with a primary distinction: The equivalence trial does not reflect the one-sided perspective of the noninferiority hypothesis. A one-sided hypothesis is one that is examining changes in one direction only, such as improvement in the measured clinical outcome; a two-sided hypothesis is one that examines change in either direction.

For a noninferiority trial (in which values less than the null value 1 favor the new therapy), the upper bound of the CI for the treatment difference must be lower than a *prespecified* minimum value. The question then is whether the investigators establish and report, prior to the analysis, the upper bound of the CI that would be accepted as clinical noninferiority. On the basis of data in the POSITIVE trial scenario, the upper limit for noninferiority was set at 1.1.

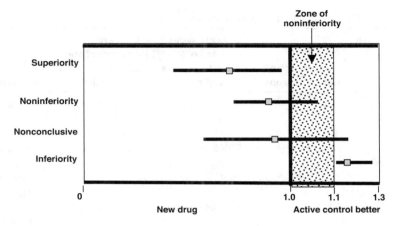

Figure 4–3

Boundaries used in noninferiority trials often used to compare new drugs with gold standards or other active controls.

This study had the prespecified limit set by experts (i.e., the experts stated, "If the upper limit is more than 1.1, the new drug is likely inferior to the gold standard"). In Figure 4–3, the CIs (upper limits) for the noninferiority conclusion and the nonconclusive examples show that both examples are not statistically significantly different from the standard therapy (their CIs both include 1). The upper limit being greater than 1.1 in the nonconclusive example means that the new therapy could not be considered noninferior, but neither is it clearly inferior.

Statistical Methods

There has been considerable debate for several years regarding the relative merits of *P* values versus CIs. The bottom line is that they both matter. The *P* value clearly lets us know the likelihood of any observation occurring by chance alone. The investigator should not simply report that "the finding was statistically significant at an alpha level of .05," but should report exactly how significant. For example, a report of "$P = .047$" is not nearly as reassuring as "$P = .015$" in terms of the probability of chance being the cause of the observed effects.

Even when the probability of an observation being due to chance is extremely small, as discussed earlier, the degree of statistical significance is a function of both magnitude of effect and sample size. Similar to the children's story "Goldilocks and the Three Bears," the sample size should not be "too large" or "too small," but instead "just right." The CI provides critical information of the probable limits of the magnitude of effect, regardless of how statistically significant the observation is. For example, if the investigator has chosen a "5 mg/dL difference" to be the clinically important difference, there should be a more cautious interpretation of a CI of 5.2 to 8.4 than a CI of 7.2 to 10.4, even if both observations have very low *P* values. The *P* value and the CI provide different information, and both are important.

Statistical tests are appropriate only to the degree to which their assumptions have been met. For example, the independent *t* test is based on the assumption that samples are independent; when this assumption is violated, the two-sample unpaired *t* test is not appropriate, and the results of the analysis may be incorrect or misleading. If the assumption of normality is violated or if outliers are present, the *t* test may not be the most powerful test, which could influence the study's ability to detect a true difference. If the *population variances* are not

Table 4–3   Matching Data With the Appropriate Statistical Tests

Goal	Data are normal and continuous*	Data are skewed, or data are discrete, or data are ordinal	Data are categorical and binary (two levels)	Survival data
Compare two independent samples[†]	t test	Mann–Whitney U test	Chi-square (χ^2) test (or Fisher exact test)	Log-rank or Mantel–Haenszel test
Compare two paired samples[‡]	Paired t test	Wilcoxon matched pairs test	McNemar test	Conditional proportional hazards regression model
Compare three or more independent samples	ANOVA	Kruskal–Wallis test	Chi-square (χ^2) test	Cox proportional hazards regression model
Quantify association between two variables	Pearson correlation	Spearman correlation	Contingency coefficients	
Predict value from another measured variable	Simple linear regression or nonlinear regression analysis	Nonparametric regression analysis	Simple logistic regression analysis	Cox proportional hazards regression model

ANOVA = Analysis of variance.

* If the assumption in a parametric test is proven not to be true, the researcher must use a nonparametric test that is equivalent to the parametric test (e.g., Mann–Whitney U test for the t test) for the difference being tested.

[†] Samples are "independent" when they are not related to each other. For example, the mean cholesterol level of the group receiving drug A is "independent" of the mean cholesterol level of the group receiving drug B.

[‡] Paired samples are not independent. For example, the mean cholesterol value at posttest of the group receiving drug A is dependent (or at least, not entirely independent) of the mean cholesterol value at pretest for the same group receiving drug A.

equal, an alternative test statistic might be a better choice than the independent t test. When reviewing evidence, one should always question the choice of statistical test with respect to the assumptions underlying that test. As a general rule of thumb, small or unbalanced sample sizes increase the vulnerability of a study to violations of statistical test assumptions.

The chi-square test statistic is frequently used in the analysis of categorical data in health care research. The "standard" chi-square test statistic should not be used when the *expected* (not *observed*) cell frequencies are small. There is debate as to what constitutes small; typically the debate centers on the values "2" and "5." A general rule of thumb is that (1) when *any* expected cell frequency is 2 or less, or (2) when *more than half* of the expected cell frequencies are less than 5, the data should be analyzed by using the Fisher exact test. When the categorical data are presented in a table larger than a 2 × 2 and expected cell frequencies are small, one might consider collapsing categories (when this makes sense "theoretically") as a way to increase the expected cell frequencies.

There are far more statistical tests than those presented here. Table 4–3 provides an example of many tables/algorithms that exist for choosing an appropriate parametric or nonparametric statistical test, or for determining if the appropriate test was used as reported in a research article. Expanded and more complete tables can be found in most statistical texts.

Conclusion

Statistics is about probability and, with respect to making clinical decisions, it is about minimizing the likelihood of making a poor clinical decision. Statistics *do not* make the decision for clinicians; they *use* statistics to help make the best decision possible given the available evidence and their best judgment based on experience with *their* patients.

The Bottom Line

- ➤ Practitioners may know more about statistics than they thought—and perhaps as much as the researcher who is reporting the results.
- ➤ When reviewing results, ask the following questions:
  —Did the researcher use the appropriate statistical measures and the correct statistical test?
  —Did the researcher use an appropriate alpha level and adjust for multiple comparisons?
  —Did the researcher report the *P* value, CI, *and* the prediction interval?
  —Does the prediction interval (even if you have to estimate it using the rule of thumb provided) change your mind about the study results on the basis of the reported CI?
  —Is the substantive effect important enough to warrant changing practice?

APPENDIX 4–A
GLOSSARY OF STATISTICAL TERMS

Analysis of variance (ANOVA) model: An extension of the basic regression model that uses categorical independent variable(s) (e.g., race) rather than continuous (e.g., age) and that compares differences in means between the various categories of the independent variable(s).

Bivariate relationship: Relationship between two variables.

Categorical variables: Variables whose numeric values represent categories, not true numbers. For example, gender is a categorical variable even though race data may be collected as 1 = white, 2 = black, 3 = Hispanic, and gender is a categorical variable. Binary categorical variables are also called dichotomous variables.

Central tendency (points of reference): Value representative of the typical or middle value of an ordered array of data; statistical measures include mean, median, and mode statistical measures.

Confidence interval (CI): Possible range of values for the mean.

Continuous data: Numbers that can always be divided (e.g., between 5'6" *and* 5'7", there is 5'6½", etc.).

Correlation coefficient: A measure of the degree to which two variables covary, that is, the degree to which one variable changes when the other changes.

Dispersion (points of departure): Characteristic of an ordered array of data that describes the spread of the data; statistical measures include variance, standard deviation, range, and interquartile range.

Fishing expedition: Examination of data in as many ways as possible, thus increasing the chances of finding something significant. A fishing expedition is often intentional, but can occur unintentionally when the researcher is conducting multiple tests and fails to adjust the alpha levels accordingly.

Interquartile range: Difference between the 75th and 25th percentile values of the observed data.

Mean: Simple average of a set of data.

Median: Middle value of an ordered array of data (the value at the 50th percentile).

Mode: Value that occurs most frequently unless two values occur equally most often; then there are two modes (bimodal).

Multiple regression analysis: An analysis including two or more independent variables in the regression equation (also called the regression model). The procedure is repeated until the best prediction model is produced (on the basis of the percent of variance explained by the regression model, or the coefficient of determination [r^2] statistic, which ranges from 0 to 1).

Multivariate relationship: Relationship between three or more variables.

Nonparametric tests: Statistical tests used for data that do not have a normal distribution (e.g., Kruskal–Wallis test).

Ordinal data: Numbers that, when ordered, one can be described as larger or smaller than the adjacent value, but statements such as the following cannot be made: The difference between 2 and 3 is the same as the difference between 5 and 6; 6 is simply greater than 5 and 3 is greater than 2.

Pair-wise comparisons: Comparisons between pairs of groupings (e.g., in an ANOVA, three race categories [white, black, other] produce three pair-wise comparisons [white to black; white to other; and black to other]).

Parameter: A population characteristic, such as the population mean and population SD; a statistic is the value of the same characteristics (mean, SD) but for the sample that is taken from the population.

Parametric tests (*t* test, F test, etc.): Tests based on certain assumptions being true (e.g., "data are normally distributed").

Percentile: A method for separating an ordered array of data into equal proportions. For example, the ordered array of data can be grouped by those in the first 25th percentile (0%–25% of the data), the second 25th percentile (26%–50%), etc.

Power of a statistical test: Ability of test to detect a specified relationship. Power is directly related to sample size; studies that are not statistically significant are sometimes the result of too small of a sample size (power) to detect the observed effect.

Prediction interval: Possible population (range) of values that an individual can have; prediction intervals are wider than CIs.

Regression analysis: A method for describing how well one variable (X) predicts a second variable (Y). Linear regression is represented by the equation for a straight line: $Y = a + bX$, where Y is the dependent variable, a is the point where the straight line crosses the Y-axis, b is the slope of the straight line, and X is the independent variable. There are many extensions of the basic regression model including nonlinear relationships.

Standard deviation (SD): A measure of dispersion used to describe the spread of data when the measure of central tendency is the mean. Generally, a normally distributed array of data will be 6 SDs wide, 3 SDs on either side of the mean.

Statistical significance: An instance in which an observation is not likely to have occurred by chance alone. The researcher must determine the criteria for significance (the significance level), or the alpha level, such as .05. For any given statistical test and a set of data, there is but one P value, and this value is the probability associated with the observation "how extreme is the value?" When this value is less than the prestated alpha level, the test is declared statistically significant.

Statistical test: Mathematical procedure for determining the likelihood of an event (i.e., likelihood it is due to chance alone).

Stepwise procedure: Procedure for how multiple independent variables are entered into the regression equation for analysis. In a "forward stepwise" procedure, one variable is entered at a time, while in a "backward stepwise" procedure, all variables are entered at once and then taken out one at a time.

Substantive, practical, or clinical significance: Importance of an observation from a practical or clinical perspective. For example, a decrease of total cholesterol of 2 mg/dL may be statistically significant, but it has little clinical value.

t **test:** Parametric statistical test used to compare differences between continuous data (e.g., two means).

Type I error: Probability of incorrectly rejecting the null hypothesis (i.e., concluding the null hypothesis is incorrect when, in fact, it is correct). Type I error is equal to the significance or alpha level.

Type II error: Probability of incorrectly failing to reject the null hypothesis (i.e., concluding the null hypothesis is correct when, in fact, it is incorrect). Type II error is equal to the beta level, and the power of the test is equal to 1 minus beta. Type I and type II errors are inversely related: As one decreases, the other increases.

Univariate analysis: Analysis or exploration of one variable at a time, and not in relation to any other variable. A univariate question would be "what is the average age?" A nonunivariate question would be "what is the average age of women and the average age of men?" The two variables being studied by the second question are age and gender.

Variance: The mean of the squared distances from data points to the statistical mean, that is, the sum of all $(x - \mu)^2$, where x is the value of a data point and μ is the mean, divided by the number of data points.

APPENDIX 4–B
APPLY YOUR STATISTICAL SKILLS

Web Tutorials

➤ An excellent book and Web-based tutorial for statistics is *Medical Statistics at a Glance,* by Aviva Petrie and Caroline Sabin, Blackwell Science LTD, 2004; http://www.medstatsaag.com is the online companion. This text is part of a series famous for its practical layout, concise text, and clear conceptual diagrams. Each chapter covers one essential topic and usually is no more than two pages.

➤ An Excel spreadsheet to calculate 95% CIs can be downloaded from the Centre for Evidence-Based Medicine Web site at http://www.cebm.net; select "downloads" under "teaching EBM."

Additional Reading

➤ Greenhalgh T. Statistics for the non-statistician, I. Different types of data need different statistical tests. *BMJ.* 1997;315:364–6. Available for free at: http://bmj.bmjjournals.com/cgi/content/full/315/7104/364.

➤ Greenhalgh T. Statistics for the non-statistician, II. "Significant" relations and their pitfalls. *BMJ.* 1997;315:422–5. Available for free at: http://bmj.bmjjournals.com/archive/710/7105ed.htm.

Exercises

Scenario 1

In a randomized crossover trial, subjects are assigned in a random order to drug A or drug B for 2 months with a 2-week washout period between treatments. The investigators are evaluating the effect of the two drugs on first-phase insulin secretion. Is the outcome continuous, categorical, or ordinal? Are the subjects representing a paired or independent sample? Would a paired *t* test be an appropriate statistical method to analyze the results?

Scenario 2

Drug A compared with placebo increases the survival to hospital discharge from 6% to 10% in a study that contained 200 adults with congestive heart failure in each treatment group. Using these data, complete the table below. You may refer to the following Web site: http://www.healthcare.ubc.ca/calc/clinsig.html.

Control event rate		
Experimental event rate		
Absolute risk reduction		95% CI
Number needed to treat		
Relative risk reduction		95% CI

TRANSFORMING EVIDENCE
INTO ACTION

Elaine Chiquette

ONCE ALL STUDIES ARE GATHERED, those addressing other questions are eliminated, and only those trials with the best methods remain, one question remains: So what? Also known as the "who cares" test, applying this admittedly crude criterion begins the process of asking oneself, "Will these findings change the way I will treat or prevent this disease in my practice—and specifically for the patient sitting in front of me right now?"

Interpreting evidence requires knowledge of methodology (see Chapter 3) and statistics (see Chapter 4). Transforming evidence into practice requires combining the best evidence with knowledge of disease and patient management. It may be the best available evidence, but the clinician must decide whether it makes a difference for specific patients.

The first step in making this decision—in transforming the evidence into action—is to consider the clinical value of the outcomes reported (outcomes are events such as death, surgery, stroke, or myocardial infarction).

Outcomes That Matter

The term *Patient-Oriented Evidence that Matters* (POEMs) was coined by Allen Shaughnessy (http://www.infopoems.com) and his colleagues. POEMs describes evidence that addresses outcomes that make a difference in patients' lives: outcomes such as morbidity, quality of life, and mortality.[1] (Morbidity comprises outcomes that describe unhealthy states that can affect quality of life, such as angina, pain, congestive heart failure, and diabetes. Comorbidity is the presence of one or more additional diseases in a patient or study participant in addition to the disease of primary interest or inquiry.)

POEMs is likely to change clinical practice. For example, the outcomes that matter in an antihypertensive trial are decreases in fatal and nonfatal stroke, and heart attacks. Whether the antihypertensive drug decreased blood pressure and/or albuminuria is of interest, but really what matters is whether, after taking this drug, the patient is more likely to live a longer, healthier life. The outcome that matters in a pneumonia trial is whether the patient survives the infection after the treatment, rather than the number of bacteria present in body samples before and after treatment.

Outcomes that matter all depend on the perspective: Some outcomes matter in hospital-oriented analyses, while a different set of outcomes may matter from a patient-oriented or payer-oriented perspective.

⌒
Scenario
⌒

You were asked to participate in a task force to review the economic impact of drug-eluting stents (DESs). DESs have been in very high demand, and are preferred by cardiologist–interventionalists and their patients. Trials have demonstrated improvements in restenosis rates compared with bare metal stents (BMSs), but really no difference in mortality or incidence of myocardial infarction.

Under most circumstances, introduction of a new technology with demonstrable clinical advantages (reduced restenosis) and no apparent additional adverse effects would be expected to replace rapidly the previous technologies in your private hospital. However, DES availability raises substantial economic questions regarding the financial consequences of total substitution of this product for the much less expensive BMSs. You shared with the group the meta-analysis that you found in your MEDLINE search published in *Lancet*: Babapulle MN, Joseph L, Belisle P, et al. A hierarchical Bayesian meta-analysis of randomised clinical trials of drug-eluting stents. *Lancet*. 2004;364(9434):583–91. The pooled mortality rates were low for both DESs and BMSs with no evidence of any difference between them (odds ratio [OR], 1.11; 95% CI, 0.61–2.06). Pooled rates of myocardial infarction showed no between-group difference (OR, 0.92; 95% CI, 0.65–1.25]). The rate of major adverse cardiac events was 7.8% with DES and 16.4% with BMS (OR, 0.42; 95% CI, 0.32–0.53), and the angiographic restenosis rates were also lower for DES (8.9% vs. 29.3%; OR, 0.18; 95% CI, 0.06–0.40).

In this example, one of the main differences between the two products is the restenosis rate. Restenosis implies that the patient, usually within 6 months of the intervention, will experience recurrence of angina symptoms and will require a subsequent hospitalization to reopen the vessel. The hospital perspective is that the cost of DES is too high. However, the payer may have an interest in reducing the number of hospitalizations. Thus, the reduction in restenosis may be the most important outcome for the payer. The patient may be most impressed by the significant reduction in major adverse cardiac events within the DES-treated group. Relative to interpreting the results of a trial, the outcome that matters is highly influenced by the perspective (e.g., patient, institution, provider, payer, society).

Surrogate Outcomes

Many trials use surrogate outcomes to indirectly measure the effect of the new drug on clinical outcomes.[2] A surrogate end point is a laboratory or physiologic measurement used as a substitute for a "hard" clinical end point such as patient quality of life, physical function, morbidity, or mortality. Cardiovascular trials use serum cholesterol levels and blood pressure reduction as surrogate end points for cardiovascular morbidity and/or mortality. Other examples are use of bone mineral density as a surrogate marker for fractures, elevated blood pressure as a marker for stroke, and carotid intima media thickness as a surrogate marker for stroke and myocardial infarction.

The value of a surrogate end point is generally established in observational studies. For example, cohort trials found that long-term reductions in serum total cholesterol levels of approximately 0.6 mmol/L (23 mg/dL) lowered the risk of coronary heart disease by approximately 30%. The association between serum cholesterol levels and coronary heart disease was

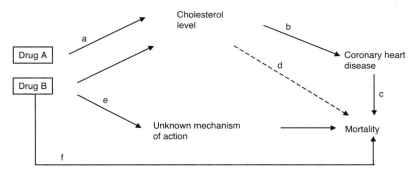

Figure 5–1
Potential pathways by which drugs can affect mortality.

maintained even after accounting for other known risk factors such as smoking, high blood pressure, and age. To strengthen the association, researchers have evaluated, in randomized controlled trials (RCTs), interventions known to reduce cholesterol. The interventions reduced the risk of coronary heart disease and death, confirming the value of cholesterol levels as a surrogate end point. Since this association was established, several lipid-lowering drugs have been approved for commercialization on the basis of their ability to lower cholesterol levels, thus supporting the assumption that this effect would translate to an improvement in morbidity and mortality.

Figure 5–1 illustrates the different pathways through which drugs can affect morbidity or mortality. Drug A is known to reduce total cholesterol levels (pathway a), and in long-term trials has been shown to decrease coronary heart disease and mortality. The mechanism for this effect is presumed to be through cholesterol lowering (pathway a leading to pathways b and c). This presumption is based on other studies showing a relationship among cholesterol lowering, coronary heart disease, and mortality. Drug B is also a lipid-lowering agent, but in long-term trials it had limited or no effect on coronary heart disease but still improved mortality (pathway d). Two possibilities can explain these observations: (1) Drug B has a direct effect on mortality independent of its effect on cholesterol (pathway f) or (2) drug B affects an unknown surrogate marker (pathway e), which in turn mediates mortality.

In another example, an angiotensin-converting enzyme (ACE) inhibitor (drug A) significantly improved exercise tolerance (pathway a) in patients with heart failure. Better exercise tolerance is associated with better clinical outcomes (pathway b), and RCTs have shown that ACE inhibitors reduce morbidity and mortality in patients with heart failure (pathways b, c, d). Milrinone (Primacor—sanofi-aventis) (drug B), an antiarrhythmic agent that has been removed from the market, improved exercise tolerance in patients with heart failure. However, in an RCT, milrinone increased mortality (pathway e or f).[3]

The message from the previous examples is a simple one: Surrogate markers can be misleading. Furthermore, clinicians often must make long-term treatment decisions on the basis of short-term trials that include only surrogate outcomes. For example, most of the drugs available for type 2 diabetes were approved on the basis of the drug's ability to reduce glycosylated hemoglobin (A1c) for 6 months or less. Whether this improvement in a surrogate marker for a short time translates into reduced morbidity associated with type 2 diabetes is thus unknown.

Combining Outcomes

~
Scenario
~

You pulled the "MUCH BETTER" trial, a randomized, double-blind study of 3000 patients with one of two types of acute coronary syndromes—unstable angina or non–ST-segment elevation myocardial infarction—who presented within 24 hours of symptom onset. Participants were treated with either a new drug 30 mg by mouth twice daily or with an intravenous gold standard. The primary end point was the composite of death, acute myocardial infarction, or recurrent angina at 14 days.

The new drug resulted in a significant reduction of the composite end point from 19.8% to 16.6% (*P* = .02) at day 14 after admission to the study (see Table 5–1 for breakdown in risk reductions) and from 23.3% to 19.8% (*P* = .02) at day 30. The relative risk of urgent revascularization (need for coronary artery bypass or other types of percutaneous transluminal coronary angioplasty) during the 30-day study period was reduced by 16% in the new drug arm (from 32.2% to 27.0%; *P* = .001). The groups had comparable major adverse events.

Trials investigating the effect of drugs on mortality are extremely costly, requiring a large sample size and monitoring of study participants for several years.[4] To improve the efficacy of trials (i.e., increase precision with a smaller number of participants and shorter time periods), researchers often combine end points such as "death or nonfatal myocardial infarction" and "death from heart failure or hospitalization for heart failure." When two or more events are of similar importance or are part of a similar underlying pathophysiology, then combining them makes sense.

All-cause mortality is a composite end point that includes outcomes of similar importance, but may not include outcomes of similar physiology (in a statin trial, dying of a car accident differs from dying of a heart attack). Death or stroke with severe deficit is another example of a composite end point, which may be perceived by the patient as having similar clinical importance, and likely reflects a similar pathophysiology for a stroke prevention trial.

On the other hand, the combined end point "death or recurrent angina" addresses two outcomes that have significantly different importance, but could have a common underlying pathophysiology. In a study, an outcome of 20 deaths and 2 cases of recurrent angina is not comparable with 20 cases of recurrent angina and 2 deaths. Data on death and recurrent angina should be presented individually, not combined.

Another problem with composite end points is that they can be driven primarily by just one component, For instance, in the above scenario, the benefit of the new drug over the gold standard at 14 days was driven by recurrent angina because the risks of death and myocardial infarction were largely unchanged.

Table 5–1 Data for MUCH BETTER Clinical Trial

Outcome at Day 14	Gold Standard	New Drug	Odds Ratio (95% CI)
Death	2.3%	2.2%	0.98 (0.61–1.56)
Acute myocardial infarction	4.5%	3.2%	0.70 (0.48–1.01)
Recurrent angina	15.5%	12.9%	0.80 (0.65–0.98)
Composite end point	19.8%	16.6%	0.8 (0.67–0.96)

Magnitude of the Effect

In analyzing studies, a central question is "what do the numbers mean?" How does one translate an odds ratio or a relative risk into the kinds of descriptors—such as "small effect," "trivial effect," or "large effect"—that are used in the published article, news media coverage of important trials, and conversations with colleagues and patients? Is an odds ratio of 0.42 small, trivial, or large?

The effect of an intervention can be quantified in a number of ways, including through use of odds ratio, relative risk reduction, and number needed to treat. Some of these statistics are more informative than others.[5]

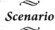

Scenario

A 59-year-old woman with diabetes and previous transient ischemic attack asks your advice about three drugs (A, B, or C). Which drug would you be willing to recommend if the following results (all statistically significant) were observed in an RCT?

➤ *The relative risk of fatal stroke was reduced 61% by drug A.*
➤ *If drug B is used for 2 years, 166 patients need to be treated to prevent 1 fatal stroke.*
➤ *Only 0.4% (17 of 4645) of patients on drug C experienced a fatal stroke compared with 1% (44 of 4652) of patients on placebo.*

If a clinician picked drug A on the basis of the above scenario, he or she was deceived by the relative risk reduction. Drugs A, B, and C are, in fact, all the same drug: ramipril (Altace—Monarch Pharma). The above statements present the same data in three different ways (relative risk reduction, number needed to treat, and absolute risk).[6]

How to Interpret the Numbers

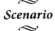

Scenario

Should clopidogrel (Plavix—Bristol-Myers Squibb) be added to the regimen of a 65-year-old man with unstable angina who is already taking aspirin to prevent death or coronary events? A literature search uncovers one relevant study: Yusuf S, Zhao F, Mehta SR, et al. Effects of clopidogrel in addition to aspirin in patients with acute coronary syndromes without ST-segment elevation. N Engl J Med. 2001;345:494–502.

In this trial 12,562 subjects with coronary syndrome were randomized to aspirin alone or aspirin plus clopidogrel; on average, the patients were followed for 9 months. The primary end point was to prevent cardiovascular death, myocardial infarction, or stroke.

The primary end point occurred in 9.3% of the subjects in the clopidogrel group and 11.4% of those in the placebo group (relative risk with clopidogrel compared with placebo, 0.80; 95% CI, 0.72–0.90; *P* < .001).

From this scenario and the raw data from the *New England Journal of Medicine* article, Table 5–2 was constructed and can be used to make several calculations[7]:

➤ The control event rate (CER) is equal to *c/c+d*, which is 719/6303 or 11.4%.
➤ The experimental event rate (EER) is equal to *a/a+b*, which is 582/6259 or 9.3%.

Table 5–2 Data for Clopidogrel Versus Placebo Trial

	Bad Outcomes	**No Bad Outcomes**	**Totals**
Experimental (clopidogrel)	a (582)	b (5677)	a+b (6259)
Control (placebo)	c (719)	d (5584)	c+d (6303)
Total	a+c (1301)	b+d (11,261)	a+b+c+d (12,562)

> ⊳ The absolute risk reduction (ARR; also called risk difference [RD], attributable relative risk, attributable risk, and attributable risk reduction) is equal to CER − EER, or (*c*/*c*+*d*) (*a*/*a*+*b*). For this example, 11.4% − 9.3% = 2.1%.
> ⊳ The relative risk (RR) is equal to EER/CER (9.3%/11.4%), which calculates to 0.816. Compared with the control, an RR of less than 1 is associated with a decreased risk, and an RR of more than 1 is associated with an increased risk.
> ⊳ The relative risk reduction (RRR) is equal to ARR/CER (2.1%/11.4%), which calculates as 18.4%. The RRR is also equal to 1 − RR (1 − 0.816 = 0.184, or 18.4%).
> ⊳ The OR is equal to (*a*/*c*)/(*b*/*d*). This is the probability for the treated subjects to develop a negative outcome relative to the probability of a control subject to develop a negative outcome. When this event is rare (less than 5% or so), the OR approximates the RR. To demonstrate this result, the reader can go back to the above examples for ramipril (in which 1% of the control group had negative outcomes) and clopidogrel (in which 11.4% of control participants had negative outcomes), set up a table like Figure 5–2, and use the table to calculate the OR and the RR.

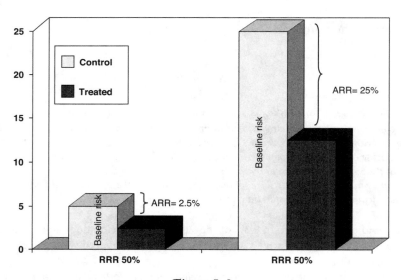

Figure 5–2

Illustration of the differences in absolute risk reduction (ARR) and relative risk reduction (RRR). In both of these situations, the RRR is 50%, yet the magnitude of the ARR is much larger for the data on the right compared with those on the left.

Relative Risk Reduction

The RRR, as a measure of the magnitude of an intervention's effect, can be misleading. It does not discriminate between large and trivial absolute differences between the control and experimental groups. For example, an intervention may result in a 50% risk reduction for the adverse outcome, and this amount of decrease would seem impressive to most clinicians, pharmacists, and patients. However, it might represent only a small difference in risk of a rare event (e.g., 5% of subjects randomized to placebo died compared with 2.5% of treated subjects) (Figure 5–2). In the previous scenario, the RRR of 61% appears clinically important, but, in fact, fatal stroke was a rare event (only 1% in the control group had an event). In contrast a 50% risk reduction in some cases reflects a much more meaningful difference, such as when 50% of placebo participants died versus 25% of subjects in the intervention group (Figure 5–2). The RRR is the same (50%), but the magnitude of the impact of the intervention is drastically different.

Thus, the information provided by the RRR is incomplete because it does not take into account the baseline risk of trial participants—that is, the percentage of participants in the control group likely to develop a negative outcome. The lower the event rate in the control group (in other words, the lower the baseline risk), the larger is the discrepancy between RRR and ARR.

Absolute Risk Reduction

An alternative to RRR is to express the magnitude of the drug effect using the ARR. This measure is simply the difference in outcome rates between the control and treatment groups (CER – EER). The ARR is more informative than the RRR because it provides a sense of (1) what would happen if the decision is not to give the new drug to the patient (i.e., the percentage of subjects receiving placebo who experience the negative event) and (2) whether the effect is clinically meaningful.

Number Needed to Treat or Harm

The number needed to treat (NNT) and the number needed to harm (NNH) are useful measures to estimate an intervention's impact and tradeoffs, and to decide whether this therapy should be implemented.[8] These measures describe the number of patients who need to be treated and the length of treatment to achieve one favorable or one harmful outcome, respectively. (Table 5–3 illustrates different NNT values for different interventions.) NNT gives us a sense of how much effort is needed to prevent one event. For example, only two patients need to be treated with the *Helicobacter pylori* triple-drug regimen in order for one patient to be free of peptic ulcer symptoms for 1 year; this example is a very low NNT. From the patient's perspective, he or she has a 1 in 2 chance to be symptom-free for 1 year after the triple-regimen treatment. Like the ARR, NNT incorporates both the baseline risk and the risk reduction from treatment. NNT is simply the inverse of the ARR: 1/ARR.

The NNT from survival analysis data is estimated by the hazard ratio with the following equation: If at some specified time, t, the survival probability in the control group is $S_c(t)$, then the survival probability in the active group is $[S_c(t)]^h$, where h is the hazard ratio comparing the treatment groups. The NNT is estimated as $NTT = 1/\{[S_c(t)]^h - S_c(t)\}$.[9] (By convention any NNTs with decimals are rounded upwards to the next whole number.)

Treatments are often associated with unwanted effects that must be balanced against the benefits. The same way that benefits are captured by the NNT, NNHs are used to express adverse events such as toxicity, adverse effects, or other harms. The NNH can be calculated in

Table 5–3 Examples of Numbers Needed to Treat (NNTs) for Various Conditions

Condition or Disorder	Intervention vs. Control	Outcome	Follow-Up Duration	Event Rates (%)		NNT (95% CI)
				CER	EER	
Nonvertebral fractures in elderly[a]	Calcium and vitamin D supplementation vs. placebo	Nonvertebral fractures	3 years	13	6	15 (8–12)
Postmenopausal women with osteoporosis[b]	Oral risedronate vs. placebo	New vertebral fractures	3 years	16	11	20 (11–111)
		Nonvertebral fractures		8	5	32 (17–250)
Patients in nursing homes[c]	Pharmacists medication reviews vs. no review	Deaths at 5–8 months (intervention phase)	8 months	9	4	17 (9–213)
Primary Care						
Head lice[d]	Pediculicides (e.g., permethrin) vs. placebo	Eradication of lice or eggs	14 days	5.9	97	2 (1–2)
Influenza[e]	Oral oseltamivir once daily vs. placebo	Laboratory-confirmed influenza-like illness	6 weeks	4.8	1.2	27 (17–59
	Oral oseltamivir twice daily vs. placebo			4.8	1.3	29 (17–69)
Cardiology						
Acute myocardial infarction[f]	Angiotensin-converting enzyme (ACE) inhibitors vs. placebo	Death	30 days	7.6	7.1	210 (125–662)
Acute myocardial infarction[g]	ACE inhibitors vs. placebo	Nonfatal heart failure	30 days	15.2	14.6	165 (111–488)
Congestive heart failure (CHF) class II–III[h]	Beta-blockers (carvedilol) vs. placebo	Death	6 months	7.8	3.2	22
CHF[i]	Spironolactone vs. placebo	Death	24 months	46	35	9 (7–16)
CHF[j]	Candesartan vs. placebo	All-cause mortality	6 weeks	25	23	46 (26–463)
Adults at high risk for cardiovascular events[k]	Ramipril vs. placebo	Myocardial infarction, stroke, and cardiovascular mortality	4 years	18	14	26 (19–43)

CER = Control event rate; EER = experimental event rate.

a Dawson-Hughes B, Harris SS, Krall EA, Dallal GE. Effect of calcium and vitamin D supplementation on bone density in men and women 65 years of age or older. *N Engl J Med.* 1974;337(10):670–6.

b Harris ST, Watts NB, Genant HK, et al. Effects of risedronate treatment on vertebral and nonvertebral fractures in women with postmenopausal osteoporosis: a randomized controlled trial. *JAMA.* 1999;282:1344–52

c Furniss L, Burns A, Craig SK, et al. Effects of a pharmacist's medication review in nursing homes. Randomised controlled trial. *Br J Psychiatry.* 2000;176:563–7

d Dodd CS. Interventions for treating headlice. Cochrane Review, 14 Jan 1999. In: *The Cochrane Library.* Oxford; Update Software.

e Hayden FG, Atmar RL, Schilling M, et al. Use of the selective oral neuraminidase inhibitor oseltamivir to prevent influenza. *N Engl J Med.* 1999;341:1336–43.

f ACE Inhibitor Myocardial Infarction Collaborative Group. Indications for ACE inhibitors in the early treatment of acute myocardial infarction: systematic overview of individual data from 100,000 patients in randomized trials. *Circulation.* 1998:97:2202–12.

g Lechat P, Packer M, Chalon S. Clinical effects of beta-adrenergic blockade in chronic heart failure: a meta-analysis of double-blind, placebo-controlled, randomized trials. *Circulation.* 1998:98:1184–91.

h Packer M, Bristow MR, Cohn JN, et al. The effect of carvedilol on morbidity and mortality in patients with chronic heart failure. U.S. Carvedilol Heart Failure Study Group. *N Engl J Med.* 1996;334:1349–55.

i Pitt B, Zannad F, Remme WJ, et al.The effect of spironolactone on morbidity and mortality in patients with severe heart failure. Randomized Aldactone Evaluation Study Investigators. *N Engl J Med.* 1999;341(10):709–17.

j Pfeffer MA, Swedberg K, Granger CB, et al. Effects of candesartan on mortality and morbidity in patients with chronic heart failure: the CHARM-Overall programme. *Lancet.* 2003;362:759–66.

k Yusuf S, Sleight P, Pogue J, et al. Effects of an angiotensin-converting-enzyme inhibitor, ramipril, on cardiovascular events in high-risk patients. The Heart Outcomes Prevention Evaluation Study Investigators. *N Engl J Med.* 2000;342:145–53.

Source: Adapted with permission from Centre for Evidence-Based Medicine Web site. Glossary of EBM terms. Available at: http://www.cebm.utoronto.ca/glossary/nntsPrint.htm#table. Accessed October 18, 2006. Copyright 2004 CEBM.

Table 5-4 Example of Numbers Needed to Treat (NNT) and Numbers Needed to Harm (NNH)

Condition or Disorder	Intervention vs. Control	Outcome	NNT (95% CI)	NNH (95% CI)
Diabetic neuropathy	Antidepressants vs. placebo (data from 16 RCTs)	> 50% reduction of pain	3.4 (2.6–4.7)	
		Minor adverse effects (dry mouth, constipation, and blurred vision)		2.7 (2.1–3.9)
		Adverse effects severe enough to cause withdrawal from a trial		17 (10–43)

Source: Data extracted from Collins SL, Moore RA, McQuay HJ, Wiffen P. Antidepressants and anticonvulsants for diabetic neuropathy and postherpetic neuralgia: a quantitative systematic review. *J Pain Symptom Manage.* 2000;20:449–58.

much the same way as the NNT by using the absolute risk increase (ARI). The ARI is the difference in adverse event rates between the control and treatment group: EER – CER. The reporting of adverse events in RCTs often varies widely and makes calculations difficult. A somewhat more objective way to assess more severe or bothersome adverse events is to focus on events that resulted in participant withdrawals from a trial. Table 5–4 illustrates one example of calculated interventions for NNT and NNH.

To calculate the NNT or NNH, the clinician needs a distinct event: A distinct event is one for which every patient can be assigned to a mutually exclusive category, such as dead or alive, cured or not cured, or had a myocardial infarction or did not have a myocardial infarction. But, in some cases, continuous variables are used in studies. With a continuous variable, an "event" can be specified by setting a cutoff value. For example, an intervention to improve glycemic control might improve the A1c over 30 weeks by 0.8% ± 0.2. One clinically relevant outcome in this situation is the proportion of subjects who achieved an A1c of 7% or lower over 30 weeks. If this information is reported in the published study or if access can be gained to the original data, one might find that 30% of subjects reached or surpassed the 7% threshold compared with only 9% in the control group. These data would allow computation of an NNT of 3. For every three patients with diabetes who received the new intervention, one would reach the goal of 7% within 30 weeks.

If the authors present data only as a mean difference, one cannot calculate NNT or NNH. Additional information such as that used above may or may not be available to facilitate such calculations.

Misuse of NNTs

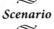

Scenario

You are being asked to review the efficacy of anticonvulsants for the treatment of partial epilepsy. You found a systematic review that included randomized trials of add-on therapy of anticonvulsants, which recruited patients with only partial epilepsy treated for at least 8 weeks. The outcome reported is the NNT to reduce by at least 50% the frequency of seizures. Drug A 1200 mg had an NNT of 8.8 (95% CI, 5.7–20), while drug B 300 mg had an NNT of 3.3 (95% CI, 2.6–4.6). Your colleague, who has read the study and often is paid to present lectures by the pharmaceutical company making drug B, tells you that obviously drug B is superior to drug A and should be the only anticonvulsant available on the formulary.

Although NNTs are great tools for interpreting clinical effects, they also have important limitations. These measures are always based on an outcome for a specific period and population; therefore, they cannot be compared across different outcomes because patients value outcomes differently. For instance, an NNT of 15 for preventing death in a patient with cardiovascular disease differs from an NNT of 15 for preventing amputation from a patient with a diabetic foot ulcer. If we have NNTs for different interventions for the same condition (and severity) with the same outcome, then—and only then— it is appropriate to directly compare NNTs.

In the scenario above, did the subjects in the trials included in the systematic review have similar disease conditions? In other words, was the baseline risk for all the trials included for drug B similar to the baseline risk for trials included for drug A? What if the control group in drug A trials had many fewer seizures, making it more difficult to observe a 50% reduction, while the subjects included in the drug B trials were more advanced in their disease state and had much higher seizures rates, making it easier to see a difference while on treatment?

Absolute risk reduction is a function of the baseline risk; therefore, the baseline risk influences the NNT calculation. Was the drug taken for a similar length of time? The comparison is valid only when the outcome is the same and is measured during the same period, and when the studies include participants with similar conditions.

Precision of the Effect[10]

Scenario

A new weight loss drug has been launched. The drug is first in its class. In RCTs the drug-induced weight loss of –4.1 kg ± 3 (95% CI, –4.4 to –3.7) was comparable to that of diet and exercise after 6 months of therapy. In contrast, a nonprescription product for weight loss produced a weight loss of –9 kg (95% CI, –20 to –0.5) after 6 months.

The mean change in weight is just an estimate of the true effect of the drug. The true value of the average weight loss is likely to be within the range of the 95% CI. One can be confident that, when the drug is taken, 95% of the time the average weight loss (of all patients taking the drug) will range between 3.7 and 4.4 kg. But if the study were repeated 100 times, 5 of those studies should produce a mean weight change outside that range.

Precision is reflected in the CIs around the estimate of the effect. Wide CIs indicate less precise estimates of effect. The larger the trial's sample size and the greater the number of events, the smaller is the CI. A narrow CI reflects precision and less variability among participants with respect to that outcome.

In the above scenario the results from the trial of the new weight loss agent appear more precise because the CI is smaller than that for the nonprescription product. This result might be a factor of only sample size, but another explanation is that the new drug induces more consistent weight loss. Another consideration would be whether the trial of the new drug had more stringent inclusion and exclusion criteria, resulting in a more homogeneous group than in the study of the nonprescription drug. In a "positive finding" study the lower boundary of the CI should be examined carefully for clinical significance. In the example of the new drug, is an average weight loss of 3.7 kg for the 200 subjects tested in the trial enough to balance possible adverse events? While presenting the study information to an individual patient, the clinician should note that the lower limit of the prediction interval provides the worst-case scenario. (A prediction interval predicts the range of values that a single individual could experience with the drug. Although prediction intervals are not generally used in evidence-based medicine, they are presented here to offer an additional view of the wide range of results possible in response to a drug therapy.) In this case, the prediction interval is –10 to +1.8 kg. From the patient's perspective, this result translates as follows: In this trial, 95% of the individual participants had a weight change ranging from a loss of as much as 10 kg to a weight gain of up to 1.8 kg weight, and the majority of patients lost weight.

In a "negative finding" study, the upper boundary of the CI and the prediction interval should be examined carefully. If the upper boundary value is lower than what one would consider clinically relevant, then the clinician should not change his or her practice on the basis of the trial's results.

The NNT is also only a point estimate; the true value is likely within 95% of the ARR. To calculate the 95% CI around the NNT, one simply inverts the lower and upper limits of the ARR 95% CI. If the ARR is not statistically significant, there is no point in calculating NNT or its 95% CI.

External Validity[11]

For health care professionals, the ultimate test of which studies are important and which are not comes down to the decision of whether to consider a study's evidence when deciding how to treat an individual patient. Thus, clinical judgment is crucial in assessing the importance of drug-therapy evidence. External validity addresses the applicability of the study results to a patient by addressing two main questions: Is the patient similar to the participants studied, and is the intervention feasible in this case when one considers the patient's economic status, likelihood to adhere to treatment, and other such factors?

Variation in Baseline Risk

Scenario

A 35-year-old man diagnosed with dyslipidemia recently began treatment with a statin. He asks you what benefits statins have beyond lowering his cholesterol. Can this drug prevent him from having a heart attack, as his dad had years ago? You go on the Internet and calculate the patient's cardiovascular risk using the National Cholesterol Education Program calculator, available on the Web site of the National Institutes of Health (http://www.nih.gov). His risk of developing cardiovascular disease within the next 10 years is 2%. Knowing his family history, you suspect that his risk may, in fact, be higher. His physician prescribed pravastatin (various manufacturers). You recall from the West of Scotland Coronary Prevention Study RCT that the baseline risk (event rate in the control group) for death or nonfatal myocardial infarction was close to 8%. The use of pravastatin for 5 years resulted in an ARR of 2.4% (NNT = 42). Do you expect this man to get the same benefit?

To compare the patient described in this scenario with those in the West of Scotland Coronary Prevention Study, the clinician should ask, "Does the patient have diseases, disease stage, baseline characteristics, and prognostic factors similar to those of the trial participants?" If this patient, in fact, has a lower baseline risk than the population studied, then treatment-associated risks may outweigh any potential benefits. For example, the results of a trial assessing the mortality benefit of simvastatin (various manufacturers) in dyslipidemic men with known coronary artery disease likely would not apply to dyslipidemic women with no other coronary risk factors.

Assuming that the RRR associated with treatment is constant for all levels of risk, one can adjust the NNT according to the specific patient's risk. In the above scenario, the patient's risk is four times lower than that of the subjects included in the trial (2% risk for the patient compared with an 8% baseline risk in the trial). This finding translates into a fraction (F) of 0.25. Assuming that the treatment effect is constant over a range of baseline risk, one can divide NNT by the patient's F_T (fraction of the treatment risk). According to this adjustment, more than 80 men like this patient would need to be treated to prevent one death or nonfatal myocardial infarction. The same estimation can be done for the NNH by using the individual probability to experience an adverse event compared with the subjects included in the trial (F_H).

Treatment Feasibility in Specific Settings

Finally, if the drug has passed muster on all other counts, economic and personal factors must be evaluated: Can the patient pay for the intervention (with or without insurance coverage)? Is the patient likely to adhere to the intervention (e.g., does it require subcutaneous injections, twice-a-day dosing, taking with or without food, stopping concurrent medication that may interfere with efficacy of the new drug) to gain the benefit achieved in trials? Will the patient's own environment and the health care setting in question allow the necessary follow-up (e.g., frequent blood monitoring or frequent visits to an allied health care professional)?

Balance Sheet

In the end, what matters is the likelihood of the new intervention helping or harming the patient compared with the gold standard for prevention or treatment of the patient's disease or condition. A balance sheet that is organized like the one in Table 5–5, and that summarizes the benefits and risks of the new intervention can help the clinician quantify the risk–benefit ratio by reviewing the magnitude of benefits and risks, and by including cost and convenience.

Table 5–5 Balance Sheet Summarizing Treatment Risks and Benefits

Intervention	Efficacy	Harm	Convenience	Cost
New drug	What is the NNT? What is the patient's NNT (NNT/F_T)?	What is the NNH? What is the patient's NNH (NNH/F_H)?	Is the new drug more than, same as, or less convenient than the gold standard or available alternatives? Does it require additional visits for safety or efficacy follow-up?	What is the cost difference between the new drug and the gold standard?

The Bottom Line

- ➤ Remember to look for POEMs (Patient Oriented Evidence that Matters):
  —Mortality, morbidity, quality-of-life type outcomes
- ➤ Do not be fooled by relative risk reduction—calculate the absolute risk reduction:
  —ARR = CER – EER
- ➤ Number needed to treat is the inverse of absolute risk reduction: NNT = 1/ARR.
- ➤ Number needed to harm is the inverse of absolute risk increase: NNH = 1/ARI.
- ➤ NNT is always associated with a specific outcome for a specific length of time.
- ➤ The upper and lower limits of 95% CIs can help assess the clinical importance of results.
- ➤ Consider the prediction intervals when addressing benefits at an individual level.
- ➤ Determine whether the findings are applicable to a particular patient:
  —Calculate the patient-specific risk and adjusted NNT.
  —Calculate the patient-specific risk and adjusted NNH.
  —Balance risk, benefit, cost, and convenience.
- ➤ Construct a balance sheet.

References

1. Slawson DC, Shaughnessy AF, Bennett JH. Becoming a medical information master: feeling good about not knowing everything. *J Fam Pract.* 1994;38:505–13.

2. Bucher HC, Guyatt GH, Cook DJ, et al. Users' guides to the medical literature, XIX. Applying clinical trial results. A. How to use an article measuring the effect of an intervention on surrogate end points. Evidence-Based Medicine Working Group. *JAMA.* 1999;282:771–8.

3. Packer M, Carver JR, Rodeheffer JR, et al. Effect of oral milrinone on mortality in severe chronic heart failure. *N Engl J Med.* 1991;325:1468–75.

4. Freemantle N, Calvert M, Wood J, et al. Composite outcomes in randomized trials: greater precision but with greater uncertainty? *JAMA.* 2003;289:2554–9.

5. Fahey T, Griffiths S, Peters TJ, et al. Evidence based purchasing: understanding results of clinical trials and systematic reviews. *BMJ.* 1995;311:1056–60.

6. Bosch J, Yusuf S, Pogue J, et al. Use of ramipril in preventing stroke: double blind randomised trial. *BMJ.* 2002;324:699–702.

7. Barratt A, Wyer PC, Hatala R, et al. Tips for learners of evidence-based medicine, 1. Relative risk reduction, absolute risk reduction and number needed to treat. *CMAJ.* 2004;171(4):353–8.

8. Cook RJ, Sackett DL. The number needed to treat: a clinically useful measure of treatment effect. *BMJ.* 1995;310:452–4.

9. Altman DG, Andersen PK. Calculating the number needed to treat for trials where the outcome is time to an event. *BMJ.* 1999;319(7223):1492–5.

10. Montori VM, Kleinbart J, Newman TB, et al. Tips for learners of evidence-based medicine, 2. Measures of precision (confidence intervals). *CMAJ.* 2004;171(6):611–5.

11. Straus SE, McAlister F. Applying the results of trials and systematic reviews to our individual patients. *Evidence-Based Mental Health.* 2001;4(1):6–7.

APPENDIX 5–A
APPLY YOUR TRANSLATIONAL, INTERPRETIVE, AND DECISION-MAKING SKILLS

Web Tutorials

➤ The University of Toronto includes a worked example of number needed to treat (NNT) and multiple other NNTs for several medical fields: http://www.cebm.utoronto. ca/glossary/nntsPrint.htm.

➤ The University of Central England tutorial on EBM statistics includes worked examples on calculating relative risk reduction (RRR), absolute risk reduction (ARR), and NNT: http://www.hcc.uce.ac.uk/introtoresearch/evidence_based_practice/statistics. htm.

Exercises

Scenario 1

TC is a 65-year-old woman soon to be discharged from the hospital after experiencing her first myocardial infarction. Her past medical history includes high blood pressure (165/90 now controlled on amlodipine [Norvasc—Pfizer Inc.] 10 mg qd and lisinopril [various manufacturers] 10 mg qd), she is postmenopausal (not on hormone-replacement therapy), one brother died before age 35 of sudden death, and two sisters and one brother have had a coronary artery bypass grafting. Her total cholesterol is 260 mg/dL. According to the Scandinavian Simvastatin Survival Study (4S) trial, what are the risks/benefits of starting simvastatin (various manufacturers)?

Read the 4S trial in Randomised trial of cholesterol lowering in 4444 patients with coronary heart disease: the Scandinavian Simvastatin Survival Study (4S). *Lancet.* 1994;344(8934):1383–9, and decide whether the results apply to this patient. Use the applicability worksheet provided in this appendix.

Scenario 2

Read this randomized controlled trial: Riggs BL, Hodgson SF, O'Fallen WM, et al. Effect of fluoride treatment on fracture rate in postmenopausal women with osteoporosis. *N Engl J Med.* 1990;332:802–9.

Determine which outcome is a surrogate outcome and which one is a clinical outcome; then complete the balance sheet below.

Intervention	Efficacy	Harm	Convenience	Cost
New drug	What is the NNT? What is the patient's NNT (NNT/F_T)?	What is the number needed to harm (NNH?) What is the patient's NNH (NNH/F_H)?	Is the new drug more than, same as, or less convenient than gold standard? Does it require additional visits for safety or efficacy follow-up?	What is the cost difference between the new drug and the gold standard?

Determination of Applicability of Trial Results

➤ Complete the applicability worksheet to determine if the results of a trial apply to your practice.

Applicability of Trial Results Worksheet

Checklist	Comments
Are the patients selected similar to your patient? ➤ Consider the inclusion/exclusion criteria. ➤ Consider whether a run-in phase was done to assess compliance, efficacy, or tolerability of the study drug. ➤ How many patients screened were actually enrolled?	
Is the setting of the trial similar to your setting? ➤ Were patients recruited from university hospitals? Or specialty clinics?	
Are the baseline characteristics of the subjects randomized similarly to those of your patient? ➤ Is the severity of disease comparable? ➤ Are the comorbidities similar? ➤ Is the likelihood of adverse outcomes similar to that of your patient?	
Is the intervention similar to that in your routine practice? ➤ Is the prohibition of nontrial treatments feasible in your patient? ➤ Are the timing and administration mode of the new drug acceptable to you and your patient?	
Is the outcome relevant? ➤ Is it a surrogate outcome or clinical outcome? ➤ Does the clinical outcome matter to your patient? ➤ Are the outcomes that matter included in the composite end point? Is the composite end point's statistical significance driven mostly by the outcomes that matter?	
Are the follow-up and supportive management feasible? ➤ How often were subjects seen? ➤ Were subjects provided supportive care by additional health care providers? ➤ Was there a program for safety assessment, and is the program feasible in your setting?	

➤ Determine the magnitude of the effects:
—First establish which outcomes matter (for efficacy and safety).
—Then complete the grid.

➤ Outcome:

		Relative Risk Reduction (RRR)	Absolute Risk Reduction (ARR)	Number Needed to Treat (NNT)
CER	EER	$\dfrac{\text{CER} - \text{EER}}{\text{CER}}$	CER – EER	1/ARR

CER = Control event rate; EER = experimental event rate.
95% CI on an NNT = 1/(limits on the CI of its ARR) = $+/-1.96\sqrt{\dfrac{\text{CER}\times(1\text{-CER})}{\text{\# of control pts.}} + \dfrac{\text{EER}\times(1\text{-EER})}{\text{\# of exper. pts.}}} =$
the 95% CI around the ARR

➤ Determine applicability for efficacy:

Is your patient similar to the subjects studied? Similar disease state, comorbidities, demographics?	NNT calculated from the trial	Your patient's estimated baseline risk $(F_t)^*$	NNT for patients like yours
Baseline risk for the control group	1/ARR	Control risk/ patient's risk	NNT/F_T

* Your patient's likelihood of the event if not treated.

➤ Determine likelihood of adverse outcomes:

		Relative Risk Increase (RRI)	Absolute Risk Increase (ARI)	Number Needed to Harm (NNH)
EER	CER	$\dfrac{\text{EER} - \text{CER}}{\text{CER}}$	EER – CER	1/ARI

➤ Determine applicability for harm:

Is your patient similar to the subjects studied? Similar risk for the adverse effect?	NNH calculated from the trial	Your patient's estimated baseline risk (F_t)	NNH for patients like yours
Event rate for the control group	1/ARI	Control risk/ patient's risk	NNH/F_T

Additional notes:

6

MAKING A PHARMACOTHERAPY DECISION USING A DECISION-ANALYTIC FRAMEWORK

Matthew Sarnes

THE PREVIOUS CHAPTERS IN THIS BOOK have provided a series of steps toward evidence-based decision making. Being able to identify and obtain relevant literature, critically evaluating the methods used in the selected studies, and determining the relevant outcomes are vital to expanding one's knowledge base to make an educated, evidence-based decision. This chapter focuses on structuring the decision-making process to ensure that the most appropriate course of action is chosen to provide the optimal outcome.

Individuals make hundreds of decisions every day. Many decisions are made in a split second; others require significant thought, research, and time. The complexity of the decisions people face varies greatly, from choosing paper or plastic bags at the grocery store to determining which dosing regimen to use in a recently admitted renal failure patient. Regardless of the level of complexity, people inherently assess the available options, evaluate the perceived consequences of those options, and then decide which path to choose. Oftentimes, however, when everyday decisions are made, all of the available options are not identified, and more importantly the consequences of the available options are not evaluated completely. When the level of importance or complexity of the decision is increased, the effort and structure of the decision-making process become more rigorous (e.g., buying a house).

Decision analysis is the use of an explicit structure and systematic approach to decision making under conditions of uncertainty.[1] The origins of decision analysis can be traced back to World War II when the British used game theory, systems analysis, and operations research to determine how to distribute scarce resources (ammunitions and other supplies) to troops on the front lines. By the 1950s, the principles used during wartime were being applied to the business and medical disciplines to improve the decision-making process.[2]

Now, decision analysis is used routinely to assess the value of one medical or pharmaceutical intervention versus another. These assessments may be used to evaluate interventions on an individual patient level; however, they are more often used to evaluate population-based management strategies such as clinical treatment guidelines or disease management programs. For example, a managed care organization may have only enough resources to implement one disease management program. Therefore, they may evaluate the consequences of implementing a diabetes management program versus an asthma management or smoking cessation program. Each of the disease management programs will bring value to the members of the health plan. However, a structured process is needed to evaluate the resources needed to implement the programs, the potential outcomes of each program, and the probability of achieving those outcomes in their patient population. It may be difficult for the decision maker to determine which program will provide the most value for the money that is spent.

Many such evaluations are routinely completed by the medical community and published in the literature. In fact, there are now journals, such as *Medical Decision-making* and *Pharmacoeconomics* that focus on decision analysis and other techniques to assess the value of medical and pharmaceutical interventions. These evaluations may be published in the form of a cost-effectiveness analysis, cost-utility analysis, cost-benefit analysis, or cost-minimization analysis, depending on the outcome variables that are included and the perspective used in the decision-making process. Each of these analyses will be discussed in greater detail later in this chapter; however, at this time, the reader should realize that the structured process of decision analysis is the core to each of these types of analyses. This structured process allows the decision maker to more objectively and comprehensively evaluate the decision alternatives and to identify the option that will most likely provide the best outcome. In addition, because of its explicit nature, the process allows the primary decision maker to involve other individuals in the decision making. Each individual can contribute to the design of the decision tree, and discuss the merits and drawbacks of the various options that are identified by the group of decision makers.

Six steps are key to the process of decision analysis[3]:

1. Define the context of the decision:
   —What are the decision options?
   —Over what time frame will the consequences of the decision be evaluated (episodic, 6 months, 1 year, lifetime)?
   —Determine which perspective will be used (e.g., hospital system, patient, managed care organization). The perspective will determine which outcome metrics are valued during the decision-making process.
2. Build a decision tree:
   —A decision tree is a schematic that visually lays out the structure of the various decision options (episode of care) over the appropriate time frame. It is the tool to use for systematically thinking through the decision-making process.
3. Assign probabilities to each of the pathways in the decision tree.
4. Determine the value and outcomes for each of the defined decision pathways.
5. Select the decision option with the best outcome.
6. Test the robustness of the chosen decision option. With regard to the plausible ranges for the inputs, will the outcomes of the chosen decision arm vary significantly?

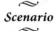

Scenario

A new antibiotic (antibiotic A) has been approved by the Food and Drug Administration with an indication for outpatient treatment of community-acquired pneumonia (CAP). A pharmacy and therapeutics (P&T) committee for a large managed care organization must determine whether to add this new antibiotic to the formulary. On the basis of clinical experience and literature evaluation, three antibiotic treatment alternatives to antibiotic A have been identified for first-line management of CAP. Antibiotic E is reserved for use in refractory CAP cases after first-line therapy has failed. If outpatient treatment with antibiotic E fails, these patients are then hospitalized for further CAP management. All patients who are hospitalized achieve a clinical cure. Table 6–1 lists the cure rates (from clinical trials), dosage regimen, cost of a course of therapy, and potential adverse effects for each of the antibiotic therapies.

Table 6–1 Example of Antibiotic Treatment Option Characteristics

	Antibiotic A	Antibiotic B	Antibiotic C	Antibiotic D	Antibiotic E
Cure rate*	94%	87%	91%	90%	85%
Frequency of adverse effect[†]	5%	10%	15%	25%	18%
Antibiotic regimen	1 dose twice daily for 7 days	1 dose once daily for 7 days	1 dose twice daily for 7 days	1 dose once daily for 7 days	1 dose once daily for 7 days
Cost of antibiotic regimen	$70	$50	$25	$20	$90

* The cure rates listed in this table represent success rates for patients who completed a full course of antibiotic therapy. They do not include patients who experienced an adverse event or dropped out of the treatment (not an intent-to-treat population).

[†] Any patient who experienced an adverse effect warranting medical attention was assumed to have been switched to an alternative antibiotic. Any patient who experienced an adverse effect that did not require medical attention was assumed to have continued with their original antibiotic prescription and completed the therapy.

Step 1. Define the Context of the Decision

Identify All Relevant Decision Alternatives

The initial step in decision analysis is identifying the relevant decision options. Clinical experience and literature evaluation typically serve as the foundation for identifying the appropriate decision alternatives.

When assessing the validity of a pharmacoeconomic study, one should consider whether all the relevant alternatives were examined (which may include a "do-nothing" strategy). The alternatives selected should be more effective than placebo and, preferably, their efficacy was tested in a randomized controlled trial. Also, the treatment gold standard for the condition should always be included as an alternative.

In the case scenario, four relevant treatment options have been identified for comparison. However, sometimes the decision alternatives are predefined by the question at hand. For example, a hospital pharmacist on an oncology service may be asked by the clinical team to evaluate two commonly used treatment regimens for colorectal cancer and to determine which regimen is most cost-effective for the service to use as the first-line agent.

Define the Time Frame of the Analysis

Next, the time frame over which the treatment options will be evaluated should be determined. This is an important step because the outcome of the decision analysis may vary greatly depending on the duration of follow-up. For example, let us assume that the two antipsychotic agents listed in Table 6–2 are being compared to determine which treatment option is more economical.

If the decision makers evaluated the two treatment options over a 6-month period, drug X is more economical than drug Y. This finding is related to the fact that reduction in hospitalization associated with drug Y (compared with drug X) is not substantial enough at 6 months to overcome drug Y's higher acquisition cost (double that of drug X).

Table 6–2   Antipsychotic Costs and Treatment Outcomes

Drugs	Rx Cost per Month	Cost per Hospitalization	6-Month Hospitalization Rate	12-Month Hospitalization Rate
Drug X	$200	$30,000	5%	15%
Drug Y	$400	$30,000	4%	5%

The cost for 6 months of treatment with each drug is calculated as follows:

$$\text{Drug X: } (6 \times \$200) + (0.05 \times \$30,000) = \$2500$$

$$\text{Drug Y: } (6 \times \$400) + (0.04 \times \$30,000) = \$3440$$

However, by 12 months, hospitalizations associated with drug Y are 3-fold lower than with drug X. The cost savings associated with this reduction in hospitalization outweighs the additional drug acquisition costs for drug Y. Therefore, drug Y is the more cost-effective treatment option over a 12-month time frame:

$$\text{Drug X: } (12 \times \$200) + (0.15 \times \$30,000) = \$6900$$

$$\text{Drug Y: } (12 \times \$400) + (0.05 \times \$30,000) = \$6300$$

As described above, because of the possible variation in outcome, a time span that is most relevant to the decision maker should be chosen for the decision analysis. For instance, if a managed care organization is trying to determine which intervention will improve its members' quality of life and reduce costs the most, then a time period that matches the average length of its members' eligibility should be chosen (i.e., on average, a member is enrolled in the health plan for 2.5 years).

Determine Which Perspective Will Be Used

The final step in defining the context of the decision process is to determine the perspective of the decision maker. The primary perspectives that may be taken include those of society, the patient, the health care provider, or the payer (Figure 6–1). The health care provider view may take the perspective of the physician, pharmacist, or nurse providing care to a patient or population, while the payer's perspective typically includes that of the insurance company, employer, or government. The societal perspective evaluates a decision in the broadest sense by measuring the consequences to a society. This viewpoint may be used when evaluating a health program or intervention for a country (e.g., the impact of implementing a vaccine program in a developing country).

The patient, payer, or provider perspectives are more commonly used. Each of these viewpoints is narrower in scope than the societal perspective and puts the primary decision maker's interests at the forefront. The decision process in each of these perspectives determines the optimal course of action solely from that viewpoint, regardless of the impact on the other players. Sometimes the decision alternative that is optimal from a patient or provider perspective may not be optimal from a payer perspective. However, given the trend toward consumer-driven health care and toward cost shifting back to the patient, the payer's and patient's perspectives are beginning to overlap significantly.

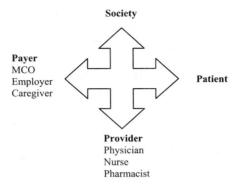

Figure 6–1
Decision analysis perspectives.

The perspective taken dictates which types of outcome variables are incorporated in the decision model. There are three main categories of outcome variables: clinical, economic, and humanistic.[4,5]

Clinical Outcomes
Clinical outcomes are the most familiar to health care professionals and are the end points traditionally measured in medical evaluation trials. Examples include such end points as response rates, cure rates, deaths avoided, and complications avoided (e.g., heart attacks, angina, diabetic nephropathy, adverse events from a medication). Clinical outcomes should be distinguished from clinical indicators that are also routinely reported in medical trials. Clinical indicators are surrogate markers of disease severity such as blood pressure, hemoglobin A1c levels, and hematocrit levels. Outcomes, as opposed to indicators, are definitive events that occur or are avoided as a result of a medical or pharmaceutical intervention.[5] Therefore, outcomes typically have a greater impact on the decision-making process; however, clinical indicators may also play a role depending on the question at hand.

Economic Outcomes
Economic outcomes are defined as the cost consequences associated with a decision alternative. These outcomes go beyond simply calculating the cost of implementing the decision alternative that is chosen (i.e., the administration and drug acquisition cost of a pharmaceutical intervention, or the cost of conducting a surgical procedure). Therefore, in the case scenario, the decision maker must factor in more than just the cost of the prescribed antibiotic. The following types of costs should be included in a decision analysis: direct medical costs, direct nonmedical costs, and indirect costs.

Direct medical costs are the costs associated with resource utilization secondary to the implementation and consequences of a treatment alternative. In the case example, direct costs would comprise the costs associated with acquisition and administration for each antibiotic, physician office visits, hospitalizations, laboratory costs for monitoring adverse events, and medical supplies or equipment.

Direct nonmedical costs relate to resources or services that are consumed because of an illness or disease, but that are nonmedical in nature (out-of-pocket expenses). For example, these include the cost of transportation to and from a medical facility, special foods that a patient may be required to eat, and family care.

Indirect costs are less commonly included in decision analysis; however, they may comprise the majority of the cost when incorporated. Indirect costs primarily relate to the loss of productivity due to a disease or medical intervention. Productivity loss may include the cost to the employee or employer for missed workdays (absenteeism), the cost to a company when their employees are sick at work and are therefore not performing at normal capacity (presenteeism), or the cost to society when a productive worker dies prematurely.

Humanistic Outcomes

Humanistic outcomes, also known as patient-reported outcomes, measure consequences of a treatment alternative through patient experiences rather than through physiologic or economic metrics. These types of outcomes play an important role in the health care decision-making process because they incorporate the psychological impact of a decision. Humanistic outcomes assess a patient's perception of the care they are receiving. Methods of measurement include validated surveys and instruments (e.g., the 36-item Short Form Health Survey, the Impact of Weight on Quality of Life questionnaire, global health-related quality of life measure, and health state preferences assessment), which assess a patient's functional status, quality of life, satisfaction with their state of health or therapy, their willingness to pay for a therapy or intervention, adherence to therapy, and their evaluation of symptom change over time.

As mentioned previously, the decision maker's perspective determines which outcome variables are included in the analysis. For example, if the decision is evaluated from the perspective of a patient with unlimited funds, the decision analysis will focus on clinical (e.g., clinical cure, life-years gained) and humanistic outcomes (e.g., quality of life during treatment, additional years of survival). Economic outcomes would generally not be included in this analysis because cost is not an issue for this patient. However, cost is often a key issue in the decision-making process; for this reason, no matter what perspective is taken, economic outcomes are typically included in the decision analysis.

Step 2. Build a Decision Tree

Once all of the treatment options are identified, the time frame of the analysis is determined, and the perspective is defined; a decision tree that maps out the possible consequences associated with each treatment option can be developed. Before drawing out the decision tree, it is generally a good practice to list all of the potential outcomes that may result from the various treatment options and then arrange them according to their timing or sequence of occurrence. For example, in the case scenario, the possible outcomes of treatment, in order of sequence, may include an adverse treatment event, cure of the infection, failure to cure the infection, and relapse or reinfection after an initial cure.

Figure 6–2 displays the skeleton of the decision tree for the case scenario. The decision tree begins with a decision node represented by a square. A decision node (also called choice node) is a point at which the provider has to make a decision or a choice between several options (which drug or clinical management strategy to implement). Per the information provided in the case scenario, there are four decision alternatives (antibiotics A, B, C, and D). Each decision alternative is denoted by a separate branch of the tree. The time frame of this decision analysis encompasses the initial course of therapy (antibiotic A, B, C or D), a second course of therapy (antibiotic E) for those patients in whom the infection does not resolve after receiving the initial antibiotic, and finally hospitalization for those patients in whom the second-line antibiotic is also ineffective. Each of these actions will also be marked by a decision node

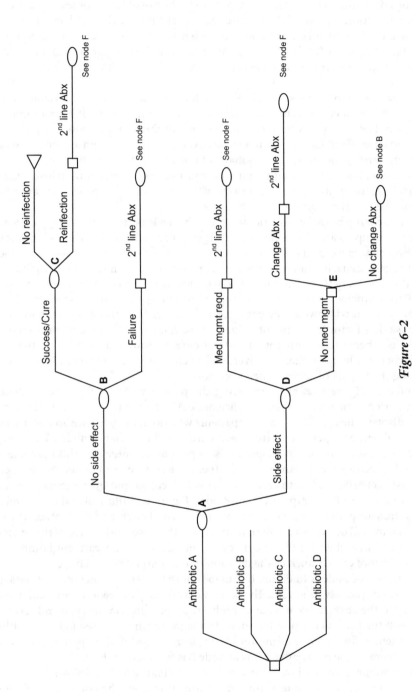

Figure 6-2

Decision tree skeleton for case presented in text.

Abx = Antibiotic; med = medical; mgmt = management; reqd = required.

(square) because prescribing of an antibiotic and admission to the hospital for CAP management are actions determined by a health care provider. The possible outcomes of these actions (cure, failure, reinfection/relapse, and adverse effects) over time are then added to the tree and demarcated by a circle, which conventionally represents a chance node. Chance nodes indicate an uncertain variable: Will there be an adverse effect to the drug or not (chance node A)? Branches of a chance node are mutually exclusive (i.e., the patient either has or does not have an adverse effect).

Once the initial decision framework is built, the decision maker should reevaluate the tree and determine whether it contains branches that are redundant or will not have an impact on the final decision. For example, after receiving any one of the four antibiotics, a patient may experience an adverse effect. Each of the potential adverse effects has a consequence associated with it; however, some of the consequences may not impact the decision, thus they should not be added to the tree. For instance, although a patient may experience mild nausea, they are likely to keep taking the antibiotic leading to a cure; therefore, this adverse effect branch would not be added to the tree structure.

In addition to deleting branches that do not affect the decision process, it may be necessary to reorganize or roll up smaller branches into a larger, more inclusive branch. Oftentimes this action is necessary because of the lack of available inputs or probabilities for more specific branches. In the case scenario, the cure rates listed are for patients who completed a full course of antibiotic therapy. Sometimes, in clinical trials, the cure rates reported are for an intent-to-treat population (includes patients who dropped out because of an adverse event). These cure rates from clinical trials would be expected to be lower than those reported in the case scenario because they factor in treatment failures for patients who stopped therapy secondary to adverse events. Therefore, if only intent-to-treat cure rates were available, the tree would need to be restructured by removing the adverse effect chance node. This revision would avoid double counting the impact of adverse effects on cure rates.

As represented in Figure 6–2, after providing the patient with the first-line antibiotic, a patient may experience an adverse event (chance node A). The top branch of the decision tree (after node A) displays the episode of care for patients who do not experience an adverse event. These patients will either experience a treatment cure or failure (chance node B). Although a patient's CAP may resolve, infection relapse is also a possibility; therefore, this outcome must be included in the decision tree (chance node C). If either a relapse or treatment failure occurs, then per the case scenario, the health care provider will decide to put the patient on antibiotic E for their second course of therapy (decision node). Figure 6–3 illustrates the continuation of the decision tree for patients once they are on their second course of antibiotics. The same outcomes of therapy will occur as a result of treatment with the second course of therapy; however, the branches will end with either a cure or hospitalization (if a treatment failure occurs again). The terminus of each branch of the decision tree is marked by a triangle.

The bottom branch of node A in Figure 6–2 maps out the potential outcomes subsequent to a patient experiencing an adverse event. The patient may or may not require medical management secondary to the adverse event (chance node D). Depending on the type and severity of the adverse event, the health care provider may decide to switch to the second-line antibiotic or advise the patient to finish the first-line antibiotic (decision node). If the patient is continued on the first-line therapy, the pathway starting at node B is followed. If the patient is switched to the second-line antibiotic, the pathway starting at node F (Figure 6–3) is followed.

The final decision tree for the one-antibiotic treatment option (the combining of Figures 6–2 and 6–3) would have 50 termini for each antibiotic, meaning that the probabilities at each node across the 50 pathways would need to be obtained from the literature. Building the most

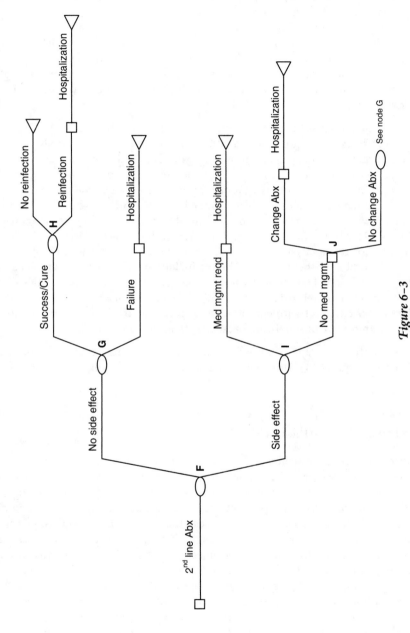

Figure 6-3

Continuation of decision tree from Figure 6-2.

Abx = Antibiotic; med = medical; mgmt = management; reqd = required.

comprehensive decision tree that maps out the episode of care for the treatment alternatives being evaluated is a good practice. This approach will help ensure that all of the consequences for the various treatment alternatives have been identified and will provide the most thorough assessment. However, as mentioned previously, the comprehensiveness of the decision analysis is often limited by the data available to be used as inputs for the tree.

On the basis of the data provided in the case scenario, we will now need to remove or condense branches of the decision tree to fit the probabilities and inputs that are available. This step involves applying assumptions, some of which may have come from clinical studies. Assessing the validity of a pharmacoeconomic study involves considering the validity of the assumptions made by the authors: Do the assumptions make sense clinically? After this assessment is completed, the following assumptions can be applied:

1. For all antibiotic therapies the rate of reinfection after an initial cure is 0%.
2. Only adverse effects that require medical attention are included in this analysis. If an adverse effect requiring medical attention was experienced, the patient was assumed to have been treated for the adverse effect that they experienced and then changed to the second-line antibiotic. Patients who may have experienced an adverse effect that did not require medical attention were grouped in the "no adverse effect" branch. These patients were assumed to have not used any direct medical resources to manage their adverse effect and to have continued on their antibiotic as prescribed.
3. The cure rates for this analysis represent success rates for patients who completed a full course of antibiotic therapy. They do not include patients who experienced an adverse event or dropped out of the treatment (not an intent-to-treat population).
4. All patients who failed their original antibiotic were placed on antibiotic E.
5. If a patient experienced a treatment failure after receiving the second-line antibiotic (antibiotic E), they were hospitalized for further treatment of their CAP.

After these assumptions are applied, the revised decision tree has seven termini for each antibiotic alternative (Figure 6–4). This tree will be used in the remaining steps of the decision analysis.

Step 3. Assign Probabilities to the Decision Pathways

Now that the decision tree is constructed, the decision maker must determine the likelihood of a patient proceeding down each treatment pathway. Probabilities for occurrence of each outcome are assigned from left to right in accordance with the flow of the decision tree. (In a real-world setting, a decision tree's flow is not applicable unless it approximates that clinician's practice.) The probabilities assigned to the branches at each node must total 100% for that node. If the total does not equal 100%, then it is likely that one of the potential consequence pathways was omitted from the tree. Because the objective of the case scenario is to choose one of the four treatment alternatives (antibiotics A, B, C, and D) to include on formulary, assignment of probabilities will be conducted for each antibiotic individually, beginning at node A.

Rarely will the authors have a randomized controlled trial that compares all of the relevant alternatives in a head-to-head fashion. The data sources will typically include several individual randomized controlled trials or systematic reviews. Therefore, the clinician must assess the validity of the data sources used by the author. Were the studies included for the analysis of good quality? The studies used must assess the utility of the drug for the condition of interest, and should include patients of similar baseline risk for positive and negative outcomes.

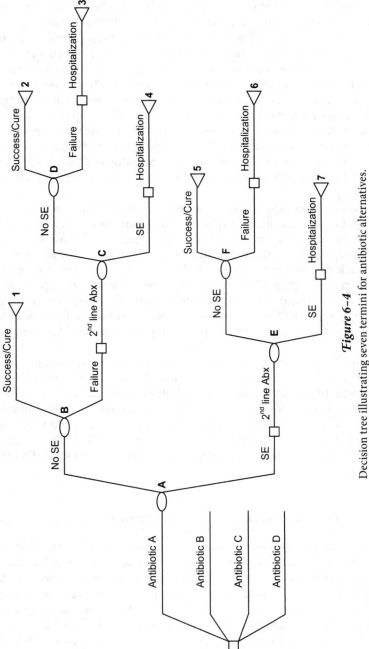

Figure 6–4

Decision tree illustrating seven termini for antibiotic alternatives.
SE = Side effect; Abx = antibiotic.

A similar critical appraisal to systematic review can be applied to pharmacoeconomic analyses because they most often pool data from several trials.

As illustrated in Figure 6–5, the probability of a patient who receives antibiotic A experiencing an adverse effect is 5%. Therefore, 0.05 is assigned to the adverse-effect branch of node A and 0.95 is assigned to the no-adverse-effect branch (total = 100%). For those patients who do not experience an adverse effect, their rate of cure after completing a full course of antibiotic A is 94%. Hence, the probabilities assigned to the cure and failure branches at node B are 0.94 and 0.06, respectively. Patients who did not experience any adverse effects from the initial antibiotic and achieved a cure are placed at the first terminus in the decision tree (pathway 1). However, patients who did not experience any adverse effects, but failed the initial antibiotic therapy, are placed on antibiotic E. Node C divides this patient population into two groups: Those who have an adverse effect from antibiotic E (18%), and those who do not (82%). Patients who did not experience any adverse effects from antibiotic E reach node D where, according to data in Table 6–1, 85% of patients achieved clinical cure (pathway 2), while 15% of patients are hospitalized (per the assumptions outlined above) because of failure on their second course of antibiotics (pathway 3).

At node C, patients who experienced an adverse effect from antibiotic E will require an additional change in antibiotic therapy. Again, per the assumptions listed for this exercise, any patient who fails their second course of antibiotics is admitted to the hospital for further CAP management; thus, patients in this group reach a terminus at the end of pathway 4.

The other branch originating from node A shows the 5% of patients who experienced an adverse effect from antibiotic A; all of these patients were assumed to require medical attention and to have been changed to the second-line antibiotic (antibiotic E). At this point in the tree, one can simply apply the probabilities from nodes C and D to nodes E and F, respectively, because both of these segments of the tree represent the consequences of treating patients with antibiotic E.

The assignment of probabilities across the decision tree is then repeated for the other three treatment alternatives. Table 6–3 lists the probabilities by pathway for each of the four antibiotic treatment alternatives. Multiplying the probabilities at each node in a given pathway identifies the percentage of the population that reaches the terminus of that respective pathway. The sum of the probabilities at the termini for all of the pathways should total 1.00 or should equal the total population that enters the decision tree. For example, if a theoretical population of 1000 patients is given antibiotic A, 893 would follow pathway 1, 40 would follow pathway 2, 7 would follow pathway 3, and so on.

Step 4. Determine the Value and Outcomes of Each Pathway

Now that the probability of a patient following each pathway has been quantified, the next step is to determine the total amount of resources that are consumed along each of the seven pathways. To accomplish this, the decision makers must first determine the resources that are consumed for each branch of the decision tree at the various nodes. The decision makers should be explicit about how they estimated resource utilization and costs so that other clinicians may determine whether they can anticipate a similar cost benefit in their setting.

Following the decision tree from left to right, the assumption is that an office visit and the respective antibiotic prescription were consumed at the initial branch for each individual treatment option. Next, if an adverse effect occurs as a result of receiving the initial antibiotic

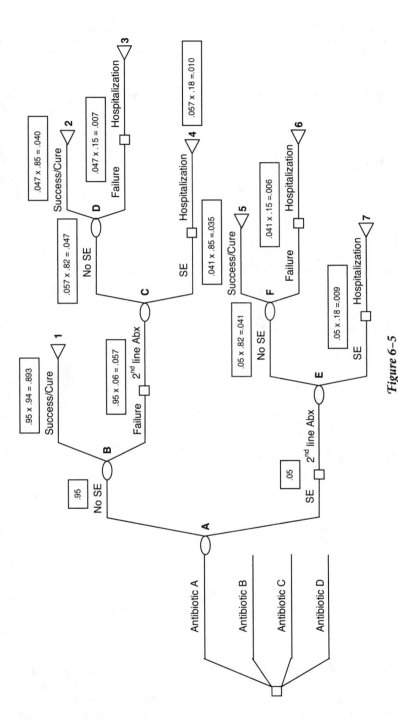

Figure 6-5

Decision tree listing probabilities for seven termini for antibiotic alternatives. (Adapted from SUNY Downstate Medical Center, Medical Research Library of Brooklyn. SUNY Downstate Medical Center Evidence-Based Tutorial Web tutorial. Available at: http:// servers.medlib.hscbklyn.edu/ebm/toc.html. Accessed October 19, 2006.) SE = Side effect; Abx = antibiotic.

Table 6–3 Assignment of Probabilities by Pathway for Each Treatment Alternative

Antibiotics	Node A	Node B	Node C	Node D	Node E	Node F	Total
Antibiotic A							
Pathway 1	.95	.94					.893
Pathway 2	.95	.06	.82	.85			.040
Pathway 3	.95	.06	.82	.15			.007
Pathway 4	.95	.06	.18				.010
Pathway 5	.05				.82	.85	.035
Pathway 6	.05				.82	.15	.006
Pathway 7	.05				.18		.009
							1.00
Antibiotic B							
Pathway 1	.90	.87					.783
Pathway 2	.90	.13	.82	.85			.082
Pathway 3	.90	.13	.82	.15			.014
Pathway 4	.90	.13	.18				.021
Pathway 5	.10				.82	.85	.070
Pathway 6	.10				.82	.15	.012
Pathway 7	.10				.18		.018
							1.00
Antibiotic C							
Pathway 1	.85	.91					.774
Pathway 2	.85	.09	.82	.85			.053
Pathway 3	.85	.09	.82	.15			.009
Pathway 4	.85	.09	.18				.014
Pathway 5	.15				.82	.85	.105
Pathway 6	.15				.82	.15	.018
Pathway 7	.15				.18		.027
							1.00
Antibiotic D							
Pathway 1	.75	.90					.675
Pathway 2	.75	.10	.82	.85			.052
Pathway 3	.75	.10	.82	.15			.009
Pathway 4	.75	.10	.18				.014
Pathway 5	.25				.82	.85	.174
Pathway 6	.25				.82	.15	.031
Pathway 7	.25				.18		.045
							1.00

prescription, another office visit is required to manage the adverse effect, and a second antibiotic prescription is given (antibiotic E). In addition, because of the adverse effect profiles for the individual antibiotics, laboratory tests are needed for some of the antibiotic therapies. Table 6–4 lists the laboratory tests and their associated costs for each of the four treatment options. These costs should also be factored into the overall cost of managing an adverse effect for each

Table 6–4   Laboratory Tests (by Antibiotic) Required for Appropriate Adverse-Effect Management

Antibiotics	Laboratory Tests	Cost
A	None	$0
B	CBC	$15
C	CBC	$15
D	CBC, LFTs	$32
E	None	$0

CBC = Complete blood cell count; LFT = liver function test.

Table 6–5   Resource Utilization and Costs by Outcomes/Branch

Branch/Outcome	Resource Utilization	Cost
Initial visit	Office visit + antibiotic prescription	Abx A: $100 + $70 = $170 Abx B: $100 + $50 = $150 Abx C: $100 + $25 = $125 Abx D: $100 + $20 = $120
Adverse effect	Office visit + lab tests + Rx for antibiotic E	Abx A: $100 + 0$ + $90 = $190 Abx B: $100 + $15 + $90 = $205 Abx C: $100 + $15 + $90 = $205 Abx D: $100 + $32 + $90 = $222
No adverse effect	No resource utilization	$0
Adverse effect after antibiotic E	Hospitalization	$15,000
Treatment success	No resource utilization	$0
Treatment failure for antibiotics A–D	Office visit + Rx for antibiotic E	$190
Treatment failure after antibiotic E	Hospitalization	$15,000

Abx = Antibiotic; Rx = prescription.

antibiotic. If an adverse effect occurs after receiving the second antibiotic prescription (antibiotic E), then per protocol the patient is hospitalized for inpatient management of CAP. The resource utilization associated with the management of the adverse effects from antibiotic E is included in the course/cost of the hospitalization. If a treatment failure occurs after the initial antibiotic, a second office visit is required during which a prescription for antibiotic E is given. If treatment failure occurs after the second-line antibiotic, hospitalization is required per the protocol (Table 6–5).

After identifying and assigning the resources that are consumed at each segment of the decision tree, the total cost of resources used across each pathway can be calculated by summing the individual segment resource costs for that pathway. The following resource equations for each of the seven pathways for antibiotic A shown in Figure 6–6 illustrate this exercise.

Pathway 1

Node A: office visit + antibiotic A
Node B: no resource utilization
Terminus 1: no resource utilization
Cost equation: $100 (office visit) + $70 (abx A) = $170

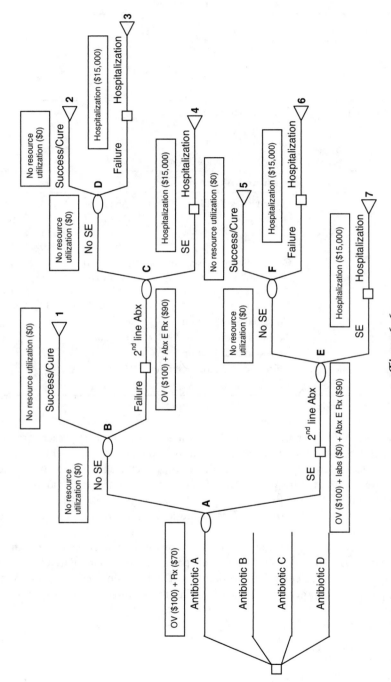

Figure 6-6

Resources consumed at each segment of decision tree.

OV = Office visit and costs; Rx = prescription; SE = side effect; Abx = antibiotic.

Pathway 2

Node A: office visit + antibiotic A
Node B: no resource utilization
Node C: office visit + antibiotic E
Node D: no resource utilization
Terminus 2: no resource utilization
Cost equation: $100 (office visit) + $70 (abx A) + $100 (office visit) + $90 (abx E) = $360

Pathway 3

Node A: office visit + antibiotic A
Node B: no resource utilization
Node C: office visit + antibiotic E
Node D: no resource utilization
Terminus 3: hospitalization
Cost equation: $100 (office visit) + $70 (abx A) + $100 (office visit) + $90 (abx E) + $15,000 (hospitalization) = $15,360

Pathway 4

Node A: office visit + antibiotic A
Node B: no resource utilization
Node C: office visit + antibiotic E
Terminus 4: hospitalization
Cost equation: $100 (office visit) + $70 (abx A) + $100 (office visit) + $90 (abx E) + $15,000 (hospitalization) = $15,360

Pathway 5

Node A: office visit + antibiotic A
Node E: office visit + antibiotic E
Node F: no resource utilization
Terminus 5: no resource utilization
Cost equation: $100 (office visit) + $70 (abx A) + $100 (office visit) + $90 (abx E) = $360

Pathway 6

Node A: office visit + antibiotic A
Node E: office visit + antibiotic E
Node F: no resource utilization
Terminus 6: hospitalization
Cost equation: $100 (office visit) + $70 (abx A) + $100 (office visit) + $90 (abx E) = $15,360

Pathway 7

Node A: office visit + antibiotic A
Node E: office visit + antibiotic E
Terminus 7: hospitalization
Cost equation: $100 (office visit) + $70 (abx A) + $100 (office visit) + $90 (abx E) = $15,360

Table 6-6   Costs Associated With Resources Utilized Along Seven Pathways (by Antibiotic)

Pathways	1	2	3	4	5	6	7
Antibiotic B	$150	$340	$15,340	$15,340	$340	$15,340	$15,340
Antibiotic C	$125	$315	$15,315	$15,315	$315	$15,315	$15,315
Antibiotic D	$120	$310	$15,310	$15,310	$310	$15,310	$15,310

The costs associated with the seven pathways for the remaining three treatment alternatives are listed in Table 6–6.

Step 5. Select the Decision Option With the Best Outcome

The patients who reach the end of each pathway experience the consequences, outcomes, and resource utilization that are associated with that pathway. Therefore, to identify the optimal treatment alternative, the probability of reaching the end of each pathway is multiplied by the sum of the outcomes from that pathway (i.e., cost of resources used in each respective pathway). Per the case example, to determine which of the four treatment alternatives should be included on the managed care organization's formulary, the decision makers will compare the sum of the clinical and economic outcomes from the seven possible pathways for each of the four treatment alternatives. The following equation may be used to determine the value of each treatment alternative:

Valuation equation: $(Pp1 \times Pc1) + (Pp2 \times Pc2) + (Pp3 \times Pc3)...+ (Pp7 \times Pc7)$,

where Pp = pathway probability and Pc = pathway cost.

Applying the values for each of the four treatment options results in the following valuation equations:

Antibiotic A:
$$(0.893 \times \$170) + (0.040 \times \$360) + (0.007 \times \$15,360) + (0.010 \times \$15,360)$$
$$+ (0.035 \times \$360) + (0.006 \times \$15,360) + (0.009 \times \$15,360) = \$670.33$$

Antibiotic B:
$$(0.783 \times \$150) + (0.082 \times \$340) + (0.014 \times \$15,340) + (0.021 \times \$15,340)$$
$$+ (0.070 \times \$340) + (0.012 \times \$15,340) + (0.018 \times \$15,340) = \$1166.23$$

Antibiotic C:
$$(0.774 \times \$125) + (0.053 \times \$315) + (0.009 \times \$15,315) + (0.014 \times \$15,315)$$
$$+ (0.105 \times \$315) + (0.018 \times \$15,315) + (0.027 \times \$15,315) = \$1187.94$$

Antibiotic D:
$$(0.675 \times \$120) + (0.052 \times \$310) + (0.009 \times \$15,310) + (0.014 \times \$15,310)$$
$$+ (0.174 \times \$310) + (0.031 \times \$15,310) + (0.045 \times \$15,310) = \$1666.75$$

Therefore, on the basis of this decision analysis, antibiotic A should be added to the formulary of the managed care organization. Despite its higher drug acquisition, the overall treatment cost associated with antibiotic A is lower than the other treatment options because of its higher cure rate and lower incidence of adverse events. If the P&T committee had based its decision solely on drug acquisition cost, they would have chosen an antibiotic that increased the overall health care costs to the managed care organization. This structured approach allowed the committee to identify all of the relevant cost drivers that are part of the episode of care for the management of CAP, and to evaluate how these drivers are impacted by the use of the four treatment options.

Step 6. Test the Robustness of the Chosen Decision Option

To ensure that the selected treatment alternative is the best option, the clinician should conduct a sensitivity analysis to test the robustness of the results. Although a thorough discussion of sensitivity analysis is beyond the scope of this chapter, there are a few commonsense concepts that can be used to fundamentally assess the robustness of the decision that is selected:

1. Identify the key drivers of the decision analysis.
2. Determine the likely range for each input.

By changing the value for individual inputs in an organized and sequential manner, the decision maker can quickly determine which inputs cause the most variation in the results that are generated from the decision analysis. For instance, in the case example, there are several input categories, such as cure rate, adverse-effect rate, drug acquisition costs, and hospitalization costs. Varying each of these categories by a substantial percentage will provide some insight as to which inputs the results are most sensitive to. As shown in Table 6–7, if we sequentially decrease each of the inputs for antibiotic A by approximately 50%, we find that the cure rate of antibiotic A has the most impact on the outcome, while drug acquisition cost has the lowest impact. Therefore, the accuracy of the cure rate inputs is a key factor in the validity of the decision analysis results.

Secondly, the decision maker should refer to the literature or another evidence-based source to determine the expected range of variation for each of the analysis inputs. Typically the upper and lower boundary of the 95% CI for each input is entered into the decision model to determine when the selected treatment option remains the optimal outcome. If the upper or lower extreme of the 95% CI for a key driver of the decision analysis causes the optimal treatment option to change, the selected decision options may need to be reevaluated.

Table 6–7   Impact of Input Value Variation

Input	Baseline Value	Revised Value	Baseline Result	Revised Result	Change
Cure rate	94%	50%	$670.33 per patient	$2654.75	$1984.42
Occurrence of adverse effect	5%	2.5%		$560.77	($109.56)
Drug acquisition cost	$70	$35		$639.08	($31.25)
Hospitalization cost	$15,000	$7500		$430.33	($240)

Application of Decision Analysis in Economic Evaluation Methodologies

As mentioned at the beginning of this chapter, decision analysis is an explicit, quantitative technique used to critically evaluate one medical or pharmaceutical intervention versus another.

Table 6–8 Economic Evaluation Methodologies

Methodology	Cost Measurement Unit	Outcome Unit
Cost-minimization	Dollars	No clinical or humanistic outcome metric; assumed to be equivalent in comparison groups
Cost-effectiveness	Dollars	Clinical metrics (life-years gained, mm Hg, HgbA1c, etc.)
Cost-utility	Dollars	Includes humanistic component (quality-adjusted life-year or other utility)
Cost-benefit	Dollars	Dollars; translated clinical differences into monetary terms

Decision analysis is used as the basis for several different types of economic evaluations. The four main types of economic analyses include: cost-minimization analysis, cost-effectiveness analysis, cost-benefit analysis, and cost-utility analysis. The question posed, the characteristics of the interventions being evaluated, the types of outcomes included in the analysis, the outcome metrics being compared, and the information available to conduct the analysis will determine which type of economic evaluation is conducted. As displayed in Table 6–8, the differentiating factor between these types of economic evaluations is the outcome unit measure used in the results metric. For example, the results of a cost-utility analysis encompass economic, humanistic, and clinical metrics (i.e., cost per quality-adjusted life-year gained), while the results of a cost-effectiveness analysis are expressed in terms of cost per clinical outcomes achieved or avoided (i.e., cost per life-year gained, or cost per millimeter of mercury reduction in blood pressure).

Cost-Minimization Analysis

Cost-minimization analysis is the simplest and most rudimentary economic evaluation method. This type of analysis is conducted only when two or more interventions, proven to have the same or similar consequences or outcomes (i.e., efficacy and safety), are being compared. The focus of this analysis is to select the alternative with the lowest cost or to minimize cost. The metric of comparison is dollars because all other outcomes are assumed to be similar. If therapeutic equivalence between the agents being compared cannot be demonstrated, then an economic evaluation method that encompasses clinical consequence as well should be utilized. The most common use for cost-minimization analyses is to compare a brand and a generic formulation of a drug. Cost minimization is also sometimes used to compare agents within the same therapeutic class or disease management intervention in the disease state. However, the agents or intervention must have demonstrated similar efficacy and safety.

Cost-Effectiveness Analysis

When two or more treatment alternatives that are not therapeutically equivalent are being evaluated, the use of cost-effectiveness analysis allows the decision maker to compare both the clinical and economic ramifications of the individual agents or interventions. Cost is generally calculated in dollars, while clinical outcomes are expressed in terms of obtaining a specific therapeutic objective. Examples of clinical outcomes may include such units as percent reduction in low-density lipoprotein levels, deaths avoided, or cures achieved. The result of a cost-effective analysis is typically expressed as a monetary value expended per clinical benefit achieved (i.e., cost per life-year gained, or cost per percent reduction in HbA1c). This type of analysis allows decision makers to compare treatment alternatives with different mechanisms of action that impact the same clinical metric. Inter- or intratherapeutic class comparison can be conducted with this type of analysis as long as the clinical metric is the same.

A cost-effective intervention is not always the lowest cost alternative. In fact, a cost-effective intervention may be more expensive; however, it provides a superior clinical benefit. For example, a population of 100 heart failure patients may be managed with two different treatment alternatives (drug A and drug B). Drug A prevents 10 deaths per year and costs $100,000 for the population per year. Drug B costs $75,000 per year, but only prevents 5 deaths in 100 heart failure patients annually. Although drug B costs $25,000 less per year, it results in 5 more deaths per year. To compare these two agents appropriately, a cost-effective ratio must be calculated for each agent. The cost-effective ratio for drug A is $10,000 per death avoided, while the cost-effective ratio for drug B is $15,000 per death avoided. Therefore, although drug B is less expensive (cost-saving), drug A is the cost-effective choice. If drug A were less expensive and of similar efficacy to drug B, then drug A would be both cost-saving and cost-effective. Moreover, if drug A is found to be less costly and superior in clinical outcomes compared with drug B, then drug A may be referred to as the dominant therapy because it is better with respect to both clinical and economic outcomes. Finally, drug A may also be considered a cost-effective therapy if it is less costly and inferior to drug B, that is, when the additional improvement in clinical outcomes achieved by drug B is deemed not to be worth the additional economic expenditure.

Generally, when comparing two or more interventions, an incremental cost-effectiveness ratio (ICER) should be calculated. This helps the decision maker put into context the difference in outcomes between the agents. (The current gold standard therapy should be used to calculate the ICER.)

The ICER is calculated by using the following equation:

ICER = (Cost of Drug A − Cost of Drug B)/(Clinical Improvement With Drug A
    − Clinical Improvement With Drug B)

Applying the values from the previously described heart failure example, the ICER of drug A would be calculated as follows:

ICER = ($100,000 − $75,000)/(10 deaths avoided − 5 deaths avoided)
    = $5000 per death avoided

Therefore, because drug A is superior but also more expensive, the additional cost per additional death avoided with drug A compared with drug B would be $5000. (It is up to the decision maker to determine whether the additional benefit is worth the additional cost.)

Cost-Benefit Analysis

Similar to a cost-effective analysis, a cost-benefit analysis incorporates both economic and clinical outcomes; however, a valuation of the clinical outcomes is conducted to convert the clinical benefit into monetary terms. Therefore, the result metric is expressed as a dollar-to-dollar ratio or as a net monetary benefit. For example, if an intervention cost $500 to implement, but results in a benefit valued at $15,000, then the cost-benefit ratio would be $30/$1, or a net benefit of $14,500. Therefore, an expenditure of $500 returned $14,500 of clinical benefit, or each dollar spent returned a clinical benefit of $30.

This type of analysis allows decision makers to compare interventions without similar clinical metrics. For example, a managed care organization may be trying to determine when to spend their money on implementing a diabetes intervention program or an asthma intervention program. Because these programs are targeted toward two different chronic disease states with clinical outcomes that are not readily comparable, a cost-benefit analysis would allow the conversion of the varying clinical outcomes to a common monetary metric. The usefulness of this type of analysis, however, depends on the validity of the method used to economically value the clinical metrics.

Cost-Utility Analysis

A cost-utility analysis allows decision makers to incorporate humanistic outcomes, such as patient preference or quality-adjusted life-years, into economic evaluations of competing programs or interventions. This type of analysis is especially relevant when comparing therapies that extend or prolong life. For example, a comparison of two theoretical chemotherapeutic agents shows that therapy A prolongs life by an average of 5 years beyond that of patients receiving therapy B. In addition, on average, patients receiving therapy A use $300,000 of health care resources over the course of treatment, while patients receiving therapy B use $250,000 of health care resources over the course of treatment. Therefore, patients receiving therapy A live an average of 5 years longer at an incremental cost of $50,000 or $10,000 per life-year gained.

However, as is often the case with chemotherapeutic agents, the quality of life experienced during the additional years of life may be reduced because of adverse effects, time spent in the hospital, and other uncomfortable occurrences or restrictions. Therefore, the quality of life should also be factored into the incremental cost-effectiveness measure and expressed in terms of cost per quality-adjusted life-year gained. This method typically reduces the duration of additional life gained because the quality of life experienced during those additional years may not be optimal. For example, if the quality of life experienced by patients receiving therapy A during the additional 5 years of life was 80% of their normal quality of life, the duration of life-years gained would be reduced by 20% to 4 years. This treatment would lead to an incremental cost of $12,500 per quality-adjusted life-year gained.

Utility measures are generally assessed through the use of surveys and other patient-reported instruments. Although useful, the utility measures collected by these instruments are considered subjective in nature; therefore, its use in the decision-making process is often questioned.

The Role of Markov Modeling

Typically, the decision trees or economic models that are built to map out the episode of care for a disease state are static, meaning they do not take into account the continuous risk of transitioning from one health state to another. For instance, for the comparison of the two antipsychotic agents in Table 6–2, risk of hospitalization was assessed at 6 and 12 months. Therefore, the decision tree would have assumed that patients transition between a health state and a state of psychosis at only 6 and 12 months, when in reality there is a continuous risk of patients slipping back into a psychotic state or recovering to a healthy state at any time point over the entire analysis period. Markov modeling attempts to simulate this reality of continuous risk by determining transitioning probabilities between health states or outcomes at frequent intervals over the evaluation period.[6] For example, the transition between a healthy state and hospitalization may be assessed on a monthly basis (rather than at only 6 and 12 months) over the 1-year period. An inherent problem with Markov modeling is the lack of data to drive the transition probabilities over the time period. Oftentimes, one must estimate the transition probabilities from the time period–defined hazard rates (i.e., 6 and 12 months rates) that are provided in clinical trials. To make these estimates, one would need to determine whether the hazard rates from the clinical trials were linear over the time period. For a detailed description of the principles of Markov models, readers should refer to text by Sonnenberg and Beck.[7]

Conclusion

The primary concept regarding decision analysis is to realize that it is a structured process that forces the decision maker to consider as many of the relevant clinical, economic, and humanistic outcomes associated with the available treatment options identified. The validity of the chosen course of action is only as good as the accuracy and relevance of the decision tree developed, and the inputs gathered for the decision-making process. (The worksheet in Appendix 6–A summarizes the process used in critical appraisal.) Because of the explicit nature of this process, a larger group of decision makers can contribute to the process, and the tree may be modified on the basis of input from the group or adapted when new or more relevant data are discovered. Decision analysis is a core competency needed to practice evidence-based medicine and can be learned/improved over time. Depending on the perspective, outcomes included, and desired metric for comparison, clinicians may use decision analysis to conduct a variety of economic evaluations. Each type of economic evaluation method (cost-benefit, cost-effectiveness, cost-minimization, and cost-utility) has a role in the practice of evidence-based medicine. The appropriate economic evaluation method should be chosen on the basis of the decision at hand.

The Bottom Line

Key elements to a decision analysis (the criteria for assessing validity of a pharmacoeconomic analysis) are as follows:

- ➤ Define the context of the decision (assess the validity of the perspectives, the options, and time frame selected).
- ➤ Build a decision tree (assess the external validity of the decision flow for relevance to one's specific practice).
- ➤ Assign probabilities to each path (assess the validity of the data sources to estimate probabilities).
- ➤ Determine the value and outcomes for each path (assess the internal and external validity of the costs assigned).
- ➤ Perform sensitivity analysis (assess the validity of the ranges selected for testing and assess the 95% CIs).

References

1. Barr JT, Schumacher GE. Chapter 8: Decision analysis and pharmacoeconomic evaluation. In: Bootman JL, Townsend RJ, McGhan WF. *Principles of Pharmacoeconomics.* 3rd ed. Cincinnati, Ohio: Harvey Whitney Books; 2005; 175–210.

2. Ledley RS, Lusted LB. Reasoning foundations of medical diagnosis. *Science.* 1959;130:9–21.

3. Weinstein MC and Fineberg HV, eds. *Clinical Decision Analysis.* Philadelphia: WB Saunders; 1980.

4. Johnson NE, Nash DB, eds. *The Role of Pharmacoeconomics in Outcomes Management.* Chicago: All American Hospital Publishing, Inc.; 1996.

5. Kozma CM, Reeder CE, Schulz RM. Economic, clinical and humanistic outcomes: A planning model for pharmacoeconomic research. *Clinical Therapeutics.* 1993;15:1121–31.

6. Drummond MF, O'Brien B, Stoddart GL, Torrance GW. *Methods for the Economic Evaluation of Health Care Programmes.* 2nd ed. Oxford Medical Publications; 1997:245–7.

7. Sonnenberg FA, Beck JR. Markov models in medical decision-making: a practical guide. *Medical Decision Making.* 1993:13:322–38.

APPENDIX 6-A
APPLY YOUR SKILLS IN PHARMACOECONOMICS

Web Tutorials and Software Programs

- ➤ University of Dundee, Scotland, United Kingdom, provides a tutorial for pharmacists on understanding pharmacoeconomics: http://www.dundee.ac.uk/memo/memoonly/PHECO0.htm.
- ➤ TreeAge is the primary software tool that is used to build decision trees and conduct decision analysis: http://www.treeage.com.
- ➤ Medical Decision Making published a tutorial in their journal called "How to perform decision analysis." It can be retrieved from their electronic archives at the following Web address: http://umg.umdnj.edu/smdm/default.asp?vol=17&num=02.

Exercises

Scenario 1

You are a member of your hospital's pharmacy and therapeutics (P&T) committee. Many of the orthopedic surgeons in your hospital have recently been submitting written requests for the addition of fondaparinux (Arixtra—GlaxoSmithKline) to the hospital formulary. Currently, enoxaparin (Lovenox—sanofi-aventis) is the only low-molecular-weight heparin approved for use in your hospital. Last week, the P&T committee met to discuss the clinical profiles of fonduparinux and enoxaparin. At the end of the meeting, the head of the P&T committee requested that you lead the effort in determining the cost impact of adding fonduparinux to the formulary. You search PubMed for cost analyses comparing the two agents and identify the following article: Sullivan SD, Davidson BL, Kahn SR, Muntz JE, et al. A cost-effectiveness analysis of fondaparinux sodium compared with enoxaparin sodium as prophylaxis against venous thromboembolism: use in patients undergoing major orthopaedic surgery. *Pharmaco-Economics*. 2004;22(9):605–20.

Read the article; then use the worksheet to decide if you believe the results.

Scenario 2

You are the infectious disease pharmacist at an academic institution. In response to the increasing prevalence of methicillin-resistant *Staphylococcus aureus* at your institution, the P&T Committee has begun evaluating whether to add linezolid (Zyvox—Pfizer Inc.) to the hospital formulary for the management of cellulitis cases. The committee has called upon your expertise to determine whether addition of linezolid not only makes clinical sense, but also makes economic sense. To assess the potential economic impact of managing cellulitis patients with linezolid in your hospital, you search PubMed to determine whether a cost analysis with relevant comparisons has been previously conducted. You find the article Vinken AG, Li JZ, Balan DA, Rittenhouse BE, et al. Comparison of linezolid with oxacillin or vancomycin in the empiric treatment of cellulitis in US hospitals. *Am J Ther*. 2003;10(4):264–74.

Read the article and decide whether you find the results convincing. Use the critical appraisal worksheet provided as a tool in this appendix.

Critical Appraisal Worksheet: For Pharmacoeconomic Analyses

Checklist	Comments
Questions addressed by the study are: ≻ Is the study relevant to your information needs? ≻ Is the economic analysis chosen the best approach (i.e., is it a cost-effectiveness, cost-benefit, cost-utility, or cost-minimization analysis)? ≻ Is it an economic assessment of a single clinical trial or from multiple sources?	
Is the viewpoint or perspective for the analysis stated clearly? ≻ Do the authors of the analysis state the perspective taken? ≻ Can you identify the perspective taken on the basis of the outcomes that are valued in the analysis? ≻ Is the viewpoint used in this analysis relevant to your practice setting? Will the perspective taken help you in your decision-making process?	
Were all the appropriate alternatives considered? ≻ Is the "do-nothing" strategy considered? ≻ Is the gold standard for therapy considered in the alternatives? ≻ Are the doses, frequency, and length of therapy reflective of your practice? ≻ Were the efficacy data for each alternative proven from randomized controlled trials? ≻ Was the efficacy data for each alternative proven in patients with similar diseases?	
What are the costs and consequences? ≻ Are all relevant outcomes—including adverse events—for each alternative identified? ≻ Are all costs and consequences relevant to the perspective selected? ≻ How did the authors determine the probabilities for the various outcomes (head-to-head clinical trial, various individual trials, observational studies)?	
How were costs ascertained? ≻ How were direct medical, direct nonmedical, and indirect costs identified? ≻ Were costs measured accurately? What were the sources to ascertain costs? ≻ Were costs discounted or inflated as appropriate?	
Was a sensitivity analysis performed? ≻ Were variables tested within a clinically relevant range of data? ≻ Does the 95% CI still include clinically relevant results?	

Critical Appraisal Worksheet: For Pharmacoeconomic Analyses (continued)

Checklist	Comments
What is the magnitude of the difference? ➤ Does one drug strongly dominate? ➤ What is the incremental cost-effectiveness ratio?	
Is the decision tree relevant to your practice? ➤ Are the decision nodes similar to your clinical management in your local practice?	
Can the outcomes be extrapolated for your patient(s)? ➤ Do your patients have baseline risks similar to those of the study patients used to simulate the decision analysis tree?	
Can you expect similar costs? ➤ Are the costs similar to those in your local practice?	

APPLYING EVIDENCE-BASED PHARMACOTHERAPY TO FORMULARY DECISIONS*

Sheri Ann Strite and Michael Stuart

T HIS CHAPTER PROVIDES INSIGHTS into how an evidence-based approach is vitally important to help inform the decisions reached by formulary managers, and pharmacy and
therapeutics (P&T) committees. Specifically, it explains (1) what a formulary system is; (2) the
advantages and disadvantages of utilizing a formulary system; (3) the qualities of an effective
system, including details about an evidence- and value-based approach; (4) how to conduct
scientific, clinical, and economic drug reviews; and (5) how to effectively—and efficiently—use
various resources available to ensure high quality of the information used to support formulary decisions. A glossary of terms is included in Appendix 7–A at the end of this chapter.

The Formulary

A formulary is a list of therapeutic agents available for caring for patients. It is also sometimes
referred to as a "preferred drug list." Formularies may also include guidance or stipulations
concerning the use of drugs. The users of a formulary are generally insurers, health care systems, or drug benefit management companies (known as pharmacy benefit managers, more
frequently referred to as "PBMs"). Formularies help manage appropriate use of therapeutic
agents and, in some instances, are also used to manage drug-related health plan insurance
benefits.

Formularies are considered to be "open" or "closed," and these terms may be somewhat
loosely applied. Essentially, the concept of whether a formulary is open or closed depends on
the restrictions. Just as it sounds, an open formulary is one in which there are no or few limitations, so it frequently may simply list drugs and their alternatives that are available for use by
a practitioner. A closed formulary is more restrictive and selectively includes agents—and may
or may not include limitations or stipulations concerning their use.

---

* Used by permission of Delfini Group, LLC.

The Formulary System

A formulary system provides for the processes for establishing and managing the formulary. Ideally, the system includes processes, tools, and structures (usually a pharmacy administration department and/or a P&T Committee) for functions such as the following:

- ➤ Evaluating and selecting drugs for formulary inclusion
- ➤ Creating educational materials regarding formulary products
- ➤ Evaluating use of the formulary products, (e.g., measuring and analyzing drug utilization, and managing the reporting of adverse events)
- ➤ Keeping up to date on changes such as new understandings about drug safety or effectiveness, changes in brand versus generic status, or the emergence of new alternatives that may provide value

Formulary System Outcomes

Evaluating drugs for formulary inclusion can result in several kinds of decisions:

- ➤ Approval or disapproval of specific agents to be included in a formulary, including any recommendations or messages to users of the formulary.
- ➤ Decisions concerning restrictions of use or exceptions. Examples include quantity or refill limits, protocols guiding use of the agents, restriction of the agent to being a "second-line therapy" for patients failing on drugs established as first-line therapies (i.e., the drugs to be used first in treating the patient), or prior authorizations (often referred to as "prior auths" or "edits") for which a clinician has to get approval before a drug can be dispensed.
- ➤ Decisions concerning equivalence or substitutability such as:
  - —Generic substitution (i.e., determining which generics can be considered equivalent to which brand-name drugs). Generic substitution involves replacing one agent with a different agent having the same chemical structure and may be done when the patent on a brand-name drug expires. Bioequivalence is frequently assumed (i.e., it is assumed that the generic agent is equivalent to the brand-name drug). In some cases the effects of other components of the generic preparation (e.g., the vehicle in a dermatologic preparation) may vary, and the outcomes may differ from those reported for the brand-name agent.
  - —Therapeutic substitution (i.e., substituting agents with different chemical structures, but with similar clinical benefits).
  - —Class effect (i.e., "equipotency," meaning deciding which agents are to be considered sufficiently similar as to be able to group them into one drug family [or "drug class"] as if they are, for all intents and purposes, clinically the same—although some other factors, such as cost, may vary).
- ➤ Decisions concerning pricing or coverage.

Formulary Development

Frequently formularies are developed by pharmacy administration departments, either working alone or in concert with a P&T committee whose role is to make formulary management decisions, along with performing other formulary management functions. Pharmacy and therapeutics committees primarily consist of physicians and clinical pharmacists, but may also include other health care professionals and administrators or organizational medical leaders. Decisions are frequently made by vote or through a "determination of findings," often with selected members specifically designated to participate in the decision-making process. Often, in practice, the actual decision making is limited strictly to physicians; however, the clinical pharmacy staff who support a P&T committee by reviewing drugs and making recommendations to the committee often play the most crucial role in the determination of formulary decisions in that P&T committees will frequently base decisions on the recommendations of the supporting clinical pharmacist staff.

These recommendations come documented as detailed reviews, analyses, and recommendations often for a single agent (i.e., monographs) or drug reviews looking at a group of drugs to assess similarities and differences. Monographs and other relevant drug review information are generally prepared by clinical pharmacists, and address such items as clinical considerations, information from the Food and Drug Administration (FDA), approved indications, applicable patient population, exclusions, efficacy, safety (including issues such as tolerability and the potential for psychological and physical dependency), dosing, drug interactions, adherence issues, cost, restrictions, and available alternatives.

Frequently P&T committees are highly reliant on these assessments as their primary, and often sole, source of information. This reliance means that it is critically important that the clinical pharmacist reviewer be extremely well versed in the concepts, methods, processes, skills, and tools that can help ensure quality formulary decisions.

Formulary Development Considerations

Formularies need to be developed with an eye to addressing the health needs of the populations served, ensuring that the formulary is complete and that selected agents represent value. Value means the sum consideration of the overall net gains and net losses in health care outcomes, patient satisfaction, clinician satisfaction, utilization, cost, and other important factors. "Other triangulation issues" is a catchall phrase for the wide array of "other important factors" that need to be considered when making formulary decisions. Examples include legal issues, liability and risk management, community standards, accreditation and regulatory requirements, public relations, and marketing. These triangulation factors can have as great an impact on formulary decisions as that of patient need, benefit, safety, and cost.

For example, in a hypothetical situation a multimillion dollar lawsuit was awarded to patient X whose complaint was that drug Y resulted in her baby having birth defects. At the time this verdict was rendered, the only evidence available was from observational studies from which cause-and-effect conclusions could not be drawn. Despite insufficient evidence to conclude that drug Y caused the birth defects, the health care providers in the city where this legal judgment was rendered elected to remove drug Y from the formulary because of legal concerns. This is an example of triangulating other important factors, along with evidence, in rendering a formulary judgment.

Another example would be that of a fully informed patient with a high-profile illness, such as a brain tumor, who is pressing for a treatment for which there is no evidence of benefit, but there are a great risk of harm and a high cost impact. Situations such as this one can result in high-profile media stories that can be very negative. In a circumstance such as this, because of a high value being placed on avoiding bad publicity, a health care system or insurer might choose to make a business decision in favor of covering the agent, fully aware that the action would set a precedent. These examples illustrate how a wide range of factors may be considered in determining overall gains and losses to reach a net view.

As stated at the outset of this chapter, an evidence-based approach is vitally important to help inform formulary decision making—so much so that considerable emphasis is dedicated to this approach in the following section, Use of Science in Clinical Decision Making. Cost and utilization are extremely important factors as well, and often play a significant role in formulary decisions. Health care expenditures in 2003 have been estimated at $1.7 trillion, which represents more than 15% of gross domestic product.[1] An estimated minimum of 20% to 50% of all prescriptions, visits, procedures, and hospitalizations in the United States are considered inappropriate as a result of overuse, underuse, nonuse, and misuse of what has been demonstrated to be effective and beneficial care.[2–4] This inappropriate care translates into hundreds of billions of dollars of waste annually. Many health care systems today are struggling financially and have extremely limited resources, which can have an impact on what services can be provided to which patients, at what cost to the patient, and of what quality. A good formulary management system has thoughtful ways of making cost and utilization part of the equation to attempt to address excessive or misapplied spending. Because poor financial management can result in the lack of provision of needed care to patients, cost also can be considered a patient "harm."

Thus, in addition to being evidence based, a formulary management process should be value based as well, triangulating all meaningful factors into the decision-making process to achieve the best outcomes by applying a net view.

Advantages and Disadvantages of Formularies and the Formulary System

There are perceived advantages and disadvantages of formularies and the formulary system. The primary objection to formularies by clinicians and patients is that formularies limit choice, and doctors may resent what they may perceive as impingements on their judgment, along with any inconvenience imposed by the restrictions and resulting administrative procedures such as prior authorization.

However, the estimates that 20% to 50% of all health care delivered is inappropriate leads some to believe that much of this inappropriate care can be attributed to the use of invalid and misleading information by health care decision makers, such as prescribers, and those making formulary decisions. This type of information can be found in even the best medical journals. The unfortunate truth is that, as of this writing, the majority of physicians, clinical pharmacists, nurses, and other health care professionals—along with many of those providing information to these practitioners, such as researchers, publishers, and other medical information content providers—lack even basic skills in being able to differentiate a good study from a poor one. This lack of critical appraisal skills even extends to many medical experts, professional medical societies, editors, reviewers, and research funders. A crucial advantage of a well-thought-out formulary is that it can help improve patient care if it has resulted from a well-designed and well-functioning formulary system, and is constructed from evidence-based principles to help assess whether scientific information is valid and whether the results of valid studies will be useful in clinical practice.

Other factors in considering the pros and cons of a formulary and a formulary management system are cost and complexity. The staffing and management of formulary administration are expensive, as is the cost of involvement of others in formulary decisions. The management of national formulary systems, for example, can result in considerable expense and complex logistics in bringing together many members from around the country on a regular basis. Despite the expenses related to the high caliber of staff needed and the labor intensiveness of this endeavor, a key advantage of having a rigorous formulary management system is that it can help achieve more optimal use of resources for the health care system as a whole.

In a review of health care for employees of King County in Washington State, a comparison of an open drug system versus a closed formulary system showed a very large and inappropriate use of drugs, especially antidepressant drugs, in the open system. The open system was managed through common strategies used by prescription benefit managers such as prior authorization, negotiated discounts, and/or rebates, which frequently are cost offsets of use that pharmacy systems receive when purchasing large quantities of drugs. In the closed system, the drugs were evaluated by using an evidence-based review process considering effectiveness, safety, need, and cost. The cost was one-third less in the closed formulary system, which was part of a health care organization with a national reputation for very high-quality health care.[5] The implications from this research are that the right structures and work processes, through a formulary system, can help improve care and achieve optimal use of resources. These structures and processes can help achieve good choices through a focus on use of the best available valid and useful evidence along with a value-centered approach, and may also include a good drug utilization review system, which continuously monitors drug usage and evaluates new evidence. Such monitoring and continuous quality improvement are hallmarks of evidence- and value-based care done correctly.

A formulary system can also *potentially* provide legal protection in setting community standards for physicians and other prescribers who use the system correctly. Prescribers might be afforded greater protection by being considered part of the norm, and if the system is successfully evidence based, they are likely to benefit because of the grounding of decisions on evidence. In these days of high risk of medical malpractice litigation, whether warranted or not, there are instances in which this kind of protection may be important, not only to practitioners of medical care but also for health care systems and the patients they serve. There are no guarantees when dealing with medical-legal issues, but a formulary system, especially one based on good use of science combined with medical appropriateness, can potentially help mitigate such risk.

The Use of Science in Clinical Decision Making

Formulary management outcomes are best accomplished by an evidence-based approach. The main purpose of science in evaluating drugs is to inform clinicians of two very important things: (1) What agent results in what outcome (i.e., cause and effect) and (2) because medicine is probabilistic, the probability that a specific outcome will occur (i.e., what number of people treated in a specific period of time will realize a particular benefit or a particular harm?). It is by effective and appropriate use of evidence-based medicine (EBM) that these questions are addressed by pharmacy administration departments and P&T committees in making decisions about which agents will be included on the formulary and under what circumstances.

An evidence-based approach means that a systematic approach has been taken to find and obtain the best available scientific evidence, and that the science used in the decision-making process has been effectively evaluated for appropriateness of study design, validity, and usefulness. Applicability is a special consideration within the usefulness evaluation.

Appropriateness of study design means that the appropriate kind of study methodology is matched to a specific type of clinical question. This approach is important because using the wrong type of study design can result in misleading information. For drug therapy, this approach means reliance upon well-done, clinically useful randomized controlled trials (RCTs)—or valid and useful systematic reviews of RCTs—because *only* RCTs can demonstrate cause and effect. (Tip: An easy way to distinguish between observational studies and true experiments, such as RCTs, is to determine whether a treatment was chosen by the patient or the physician, or whether the intervention was assigned. If treatment was chosen, the study is an observational study; if assigned, the study is an experiment.)

Validity means "closeness to truth," that is, the studies have been scrutinized to determine whether bias, confounding, and chance may possibly explain study results. These factors can invalidate a study: If there are many or major threats to validity, the study should be considered lethally flawed and should not be used for health care decisions. Many studies, while not lethally flawed, have so many threats to validity that it is uncertain what the science is informing users. As of this writing, very few research studies—regardless of where they are published—achieve an excellent grade for quality, sometimes because of poor research design, execution, or reporting. However, sometimes quality is affected by extenuating factors such as high loss to follow-up for a population that is highly mobile or as a result of ethical challenges. For example, it would be unethical to do a study in which people are randomized to smoke. Even when an investigator does his or her utmost to design a high-quality study under such challenging and limiting circumstances, the natural laws of science still prevail—and a study is only as good as it is valid and as its results are useful. A critically important point is that some research questions are impossible to answer well, if at all. The lack of good evidence-based practice as a culture, the lack of critical appraisal skills, time pressures, and the need for clinical solutions often all operate in concert to work against an objective analysis of the quality of the medical science. Because the effect of these issues is so important, they will be covered in greater detail in the discussion of evidence versus "judgments."

Usefulness means that the results will be meaningful, which includes the size of the study results and what one might expect for outcomes outside the research setting (i.e., effectiveness). Also, another important consideration is that the science be "clinically significant," meaning that it is directly found to achieve desired outcomes in things that matter to patients in five areas: morbidity, mortality, symptom relief, functioning, and health-related quality of life. Utilizing research that does not have direct proof for these outcomes can increase the risk of harms to patients as well as drive up costs and add to waste.

Applicability means the considerations and the conditions for use of an agent, which may entail determinations of how the drug will be used and for which subpopulations of patients and under what circumstances. These considerations take into account such things as likelihood of patient adherence to treatment and the patient perspective on benefits, risks, harms, cost, uncertainties, and alternatives, as examples.

It is incumbent upon clinical pharmacists to possess strong critical appraisal skills to be able to assist decision makers in selecting drugs, and in determining appropriate use of these drugs to help guide quality and value-based care for patients and for the health care systems that serve them.

The Evidence- and Value-Based Approach

An evidence- and value-based approach should be taken in all aspects of formulary management including the creation of and method of executing process steps. This process extends to establishing criteria for decision making; finding, evaluating, and synthesizing the most useful information; developing monographs or drug reviews; and managing committee deliberations and formulary adjustments.

The principal drivers of this approach are these: application of solid EBM methods, consideration of value, and a thoughtful differentiation between the two. In the section Scientific,

Clinical, and Economic Drug Review Processes, specific steps will be described in greater detail.

Application of Solid EBM Methods

The drug review process starts with a systematic search of the medical literature followed by a judicious selection process of the literature to be considered, and then entails ensuring that critical appraisal has been conducted for scientific validity (closeness to truth) and usefulness, including applicability.

Many processes are hampered by lack of skills not only in critical appraisal as mentioned earlier, but also in effective and efficient information retrieval. Pharmacists need to know which sources to search, how to perform a focused search, and how to increase or decrease the sensitivity and specificity of their search. They also can benefit from time-saving strategies, which will be discussed later in greater detail.

Consideration of Value

Potential impacts of changes in clinical practice resulting from formulary decisions are assessed as part of the decision-making process. This assessment includes health care outcomes, patient and provider satisfaction, cost and utilization, and other triangulation issues.

Differentiation Between Evidence and Nonevidentiary Considerations

The review of the evidence is separated from other considerations, such as "beliefs," cost, and other triangulation issues that need to be considered when making a judgment regarding overall clinical value.

While this differentiation may seem obvious, in our experience, it is where *many* committees or reviewers fail and is *especially* likely to occur when the research is poor or the evidence is lacking. This confusion occurs for a host of reasons including (1) widespread lack of EBM skills in those who perform and report research, and in those who read and use literature; (2) a bias toward "approved" drugs because, if they're approved, there *must* be overall value in using them; (3) cultural influences and attitudes, which include consumerism and a bias toward equating "new" with "improved"; (4) influence from "experts" (who might not, in fact, be expert); (5) sloppy, incorrect, and misleading language about evidence; (6) "rooting" for the investigator usually out of trust, respect, and goodwill; and (7) "rooting" for the intervention usually because of a hopefulness for a clinical solution addressing a need. The end result is a tangle in which the actual evidence gets lost, or is believed to be better than it is and gets misrepresented as being the basis for a conclusion when, in fact, opinion or other value considerations are actually responsible for winning the decision.

A few of these problems will be elaborated on, starting with lack of EBM skills. Frequently, Delfini Group's evidence-based training programs begin with participants being asked three basic evidence-based questions to gauge the participants' general familiarity with a few key EBM concepts. The failure rate often was very high for physicians, clinical pharmacists, and nurses at more than 70%. There was also a great incongruity between participants' expressed confidence level in their critical appraisal skills and their actual skills. The vast majority who indicated confidence in evaluating the medical literature failed two or three of the three questions. A preliminary report on these observations can be found at http://www.delfini.org/ Delfini_Pre-Test_Report_0306.pdf.

Another problem is lack of critical appraisal skills. As stated before, the vast majority of physicians lack these skills; however, physicians in specialties other than primary care (i.e., the subspecialties) are considered experts. And yet, one can only truly be considered an expert if one truly understands what will and will not work clinically. David Eddy, MD, did an illu-minating study[7] in which he framed questions for experts in all the subspecialties. Instead of getting consistent answers, within each field he got a scattergram, meaning that their answers were all over the map. If the specialists had had true expertise, their answers would have been quite consistent. Yet specialists will frequently drive formulary decisions on the basis of their opinions.

And many times these opinions will be stated as evidentiary facts. Frequently, reviewers or members will use statements such as "there is good evidence that…" when, in fact, there is no evidence: They are merely stating their opinion, or they are referencing poor or lethally flawed evidence or misusing the evidence.

The remedy for this problem is to ensure use of a very transparent process in which the evi-dence is brought to the table and reviewed. This process entails a review of the study type and a validity determination *before* looking at a study's results. (Some EBM experts actually advo-cate never looking at the results of invalid studies to help avoid being influenced by them.) The process also entails a clear understanding of the difference between the validity of a study or group of studies and the judgments made about using that evidence in conjunction with other issues, such as cost, in making formulary decisions.

The point is to understand the evidence on its own—separate from all other issues—and to understand that other considerations should be brought into the equation in light of the evi-dence only *after* the evidence is understood. In this way, one does not make the evidence seem better than it is and does not "confuse" why certain decisions are made.

Ultimately, formulary decisions may be made that are not entirely consistent with what the best available valid and useful evidence indicates. However, those decisions should be made with a full understanding of what the evidence tells us—and *why* the decisions are being made (i.e., which of the triangulation issues is weighted more heavily than the evidence). The deci-sions should be explicitly documented as such, separating evidence from the "value" consider-ation that ended up driving the decision.

Belief is a powerful thing. Beliefs will show up in a monograph or in a committee meeting in various ways. "Rooting for the investigator" can come in several forms, such as a circum-stance in which authors of a paper stated that they randomized subjects to two groups, but did not explain how they randomized. The impulse is to believe that the investigator *had to have* done this correctly, whereas the EBM approach is to downgrade the study because of the missing information. (While sometimes omissions in information are the fault of editors, a good investigator knows that readers need to see these kinds of details to evaluate the quality of the research and will work to at least succinctly report key information needed for appraisal. Missing key study details not only make it impossible to assess the quality of study methodol-ogy, but they also might be suggestive of an investigator who is not sufficiently experienced in good research techniques, which in turn may hint that other significant study flaws also exist and are not detectable through reading the article.)

Another example is investigators who make a grandiose claim. The tendency is to believe in their expertise, rather than take the EBM stance that conclusions are potentially biased and that only results of valid studies should be evaluated for conclusions. In another scenario, the investigator faces the challenge of trying to answer questions that do not easily "cooperate" with good science, as in our earlier example of the highly mobile population who will not refrain from moving around to ensure a good follow-up rate. The tendency is to "forgive" the investigator for problems beyond his or her control: After all, that investigator cannot help it that the population needed is not going to be easy to work with, right? But an EBM approach recognizes that the laws of science do not bend just because one is trying hard in the face of adversity. The research does not get "extra validity points" for being tough to do: The science is only as valid as it is!

Belief also shows up in "rooting for the intervention," as in "we have no way to cure cancer, and so the science on this new drug now looks better than it actually is," or "drug X is much cheaper than drug Y, so I want to believe the science that suggests they are equivalent."

Even those who have strong skills in EBM can get lost in the evidence-belief-value triangle. Many EBM working groups will apply an actual grade to a study after their critical review. Through its work evaluating monographs for various clinical pharmacy teams, Delfini Group has noted a strong overall tendency to "upgrade" studies. Many of the studies evaluated have been highly flawed, getting A- or B-type grades, with reviewers making conclusions about cause and effect that should not have been made because the evidence was so uncertain.

Strange but true: When Delfini Group asked a number of health care providers whether they would rather be randomized to a new intervention or to placebo—without even giving a hypothetical condition—the majority of even the most knowledgeable health care professionals stated they would hope for assignment to the intervention. This preference exists even with all the interventions that have been used and later shown to harm people and provide no benefit—and with the added considerations that most interventions carry a risk of harm, and that there is a high likelihood that most people will not benefit from an intervention at all (rare is the number needed to treat equal to 1). This observation means that most evaluators are biased in favor of the intervention. It is this kind of blanket hopefulness, favoring the intervention, that can undermine the best attempts at a truly evidence-based process. This inherent bias, coupled with clinical hopes in areas for which there are true gaps between a clinical problem and a wholesale lack of any effective solution, greatly increases the pressure to approve interventions. Under these circumstances, even some of the most hardy EBM-trained evaluators sometimes break, allowing hope to affect their assessment of the science, and render a judgment that the evidence is better than it actually is. Being aware of this tendency and building transparency into the process are key to help mitigate these influences.

Conducting scientific, clinical, and economic drug reviews entails a number of components. There are numerous ways of approaching this work. This chapter describes one method.

Scientific, Clinical, and Economic Drug Review Processes: Introduction to a Method for Applying an "Explicit" Evidence- and Value-Based Approach

Review processes sometimes need to vary depending on whether the perspective is a local one or a broader one (e.g., national). A committee that represents local concerns may have an easier time doing a cost analysis, for example, than a committee that has to consider price variability across different locations. And even for those in a similar situation, different groups have different approaches to conducting their drug reviews. Some groups expend more effort than others by doing a fairly extensive review of the literature. Other groups rely to a greater extent on others' reviews. Either method can be reasonable provided that the process results in the use of valid, useful, clinically meaningful information to support meaningful analyses and thoughtful recommendations.

A useful approach to evidence-based clinical improvement was originally inspired by David Eddy, MD, who emphasized the need for organizations to be explicit and transparent in the steps for acquiring and appraising information, and stressed the need for projecting the impacts of change before making judgments about what constitutes a clinical improvement.[6] This approach, referred to as the "explicit" evidence-based approach, was developed further under the leadership of Michael Stuart, MD, and others, at Group Health Cooperative in Seattle, Washington, a managed care system with a reputation for being of very high quality. The Delfini Group further refined this approach into a model and series of sequential tool-based process steps that are being used by some of the best providers of medical care in the country.

The following features of the Delfini Group approach will be described:

- ➢ Validity and usefulness as the informing drivers for the basis of decision making
- ➢ Patient-centeredness as the heart of the approach
- ➢ Rigor, robustness, efficiency, and transparency as the hallmarks
- ➢ Value as a deciding force, taking into account all important considerations for rendering a judgment

This process is framed by an evidence-based value model for clinical quality improvement. All too often a division is seen in the perspectives taken by health care professionals who do not take a full-system view, but become too narrowly focused on the perspectives of their particular viewpoints, and often are driven by education, history, occupation, and existing system structures in the environments in which they work. It is important to take a full-system view that is informed by the varying perspectives and talents offered by the different focuses and approaches that each discipline can offer—such as those by medical leaders, health care administrators, practicing physicians, clinical pharmacists, nurses, and others. (It is the authors' belief that the best solutions for quality and value-based medical care can come from the discipline of clinical pharmacy albeit neither author has a clinical pharmacy background.) Medical leaders and individual physicians lack time and frequently lack the robustness of skills that can be found in clinical pharmacy, which is increasingly being called upon to inform meaningful clinical decision making. For this reason, it is strategically important that clinical pharmacists be afforded a larger view into what is required for quality clinical care. They are now being trained in a discipline that can provide many of the solutions to our ailing health care system.

The model advocated in this chapter draws from varying health care disciplines and takes into account the net gains and losses from considerations of health outcomes, the patient perspective, satisfaction of clinicians and patients, and savings versus costs, along with the other considerations described earlier as other triangulation issues. This model can yield thoughtful judgments about clinical value. Clinical quality improvement is about finding and closing gaps in quality, value, and uncertainty in the health care system. This process is based on the understanding that the best available valid and useful evidence informs quality care, and that combining this evidence with a value-centered approach, along with effective implementation and measurement of clinical change, results in a system that can improve health care outcomes and improve use of resources.

Stages and Steps of Evidence- and Value-Based Clinical Improvement

The various stages of evidence- and value-based clinical improvement are as follows:

- ➢ Phase 1: Readiness
  —Readying the organization for EBM
- ➢ Phase 2: Clinical improvement project identification
  —Determining how to decide what needs improvement and how to effect improvement
- ➢ Phase 3: Clinical content
  —Determining how to decide on the clinical content for an improvement project, including examining what the evidence indicates

➤ Phase 4: Impact assessment to achieve the evidence-based value proposition
  —Identifying the evidence, then anticipating the clinical and cost impacts of change for the organization
➤ Phase 5: Creation, support, and sustainment of change
  —Determining the objective, then deciding how to create the desired change and keep it going
➤ Phase 6: Updates and improvement
  —Cycling back through phases 1–5

The specific steps in this model are taken sequentially to increase efficiency by putting first things first. Each step includes pass/fail points in an effort to ensure efficiency by helping to terminate clinical quality improvement efforts—which can be very expensive—at the earliest stage possible. This approach helps redirect resources to other efforts that are more likely to provide value.

The steps in the model are framed by the five "A's" of EBM (modified by Delfini Group, LLC [www.delfini.org] from Leung GM. Evidence-based practice revisited. *Asia Pac J Public Health.* 2001;13(2):116–21):

➤ Ask the right clinical question.
➤ Acquire information using evidence-based and efficient techniques (i.e., know what types of study designs fit the clinical question) for questions of therapy such as those faced by clinical pharmacists and P&T committees. This process entails using RCTs or well-done systematic reviews of RCTs to establish cause and effect for efficacy of interventions, and knowing how to use the best sources in the most efficient way to obtain the highest-quality information.
➤ Appraise information for validity and usefulness.
➤ Apply outcomes of these efforts to clinical care, which includes various steps discussed in Table 7–1.
➤ Apply the A's again—that is, know the importance of and methods for going through the cycle of the preceding steps again to continuously improve quality and value.

Table 7–1 outlines the specific activities within the six phases in the Evidence- and Value-based Clinical Quality Improvement model. All of these steps require the right work components, which include leadership, organizational support, well-thought-out and supported work structures and processes, clearly defined staff roles, and staff skilled in the concepts and methods of clinical quality improvement. A key component is having a set of tools to assist with performing the work in a rigorous and consistent fashion, creating clear steps for the work, and providing for good documentation—which is at the heart of transparency.

Tips for Conducting Scientific, Clinical, and Economic Drug Review

The following discussion presents practical tips for conducting reviews. Meticulous documentation of everything that goes into a review—search strategy, assumptions used, references, sources, background calculations, unit values used, and so on—is strongly advised. Documentation is important for transparency, decision support, updates, legal reviews, audits, and other needs that may arise. (While it may seem onerous at the time, recording details during the process will be less work than having to retrace the steps.)

Table 7-1   Steps in Explicit Evidence- and Value-Based Clinical Improvement Model

Ask	1. Identify significant gaps and uncertainties; identify possible projects for consideration. → Pass/fail further development of projects
Acquire	2. Search for the best available project content. Apply systematic strategies to obtain evidence; then filter evidence for strength of the study design and relevance. → Pass/fail projects depending on lack of available content
Appraise	3. Assess the amount of work needed; adapt content or develop own project from evidence available. → Pass/fail depending on ability to acquire or develop the content
	4. Unless the information is from a "trusted source," critically appraise content for validity and ensure the content is up-to-date. (Consider auditing "trusted" sources to ensure validity and clinical usefulness.) → Pass/fail invalid information
	5. Examine results of valid content and assess usefulness. → Pass/fail information that is not useful or usable
	6. Summarize and synthesize the evidence.
	7. Assess potential impacts of practice change or other change: —Create evidence-based estimates of local quality and cost outcomes. → Pass/fail —Assess potential program change (including implementation and measurement). —Perform analysis of economic and noneconomic changes, including sensitivity analyses. —Summarize and decide. → Pass/fail project if a significant gap cannot be narrowed meaningfully or closed
Apply	8. Create information, decision, and action aids; these can be for clinicians, patients, leaders, other health care staff, etc.
	9. Implement and measure success of implementation or performance, and report findings.
Apply A's again	10. Cycle back through the A's to update information and continuously improve care.

How Agents Get Selected for Review

Most organizations have a process for submitting requests to the P&T committee. Sometimes, the process requires the chief of a clinical department to verify that the clinical specialty wants the new agent considered. At other times the P&T staff pharmacists, through their scanning of the media and medical literature, request that an agent be reviewed or re-reviewed. The latter process raises the need for pharmacists to have a systematic approach to scanning the various media for signals that an agent of value (such as one that is improved, equivalent, and less costly, etc.) is or is likely to become available for clinical use.

Background Information

Once it has been determined that an agent will be considered for a formulary determination, a good start is to obtain key background information such as FDA approval status, indication, label, harms (including abuse and dependency issues), interactions, therapeutic equivalents, and other alternatives. It is also a good approach to obtain clinical background on the conditions for the specific indications.

Information on many of the above topics may be found on the FDA Web site. As of this writing, the site is huge and complex to navigate. It requires patience and persistence to find relevant information, and information is not consistently available for all agents.

Especially useful sections are Drugs@FDA (http://www.fda.gov/search/databases.html) and the Center for Drug Evaluation and Research (CDER; http://www.fda.gov/cder). CDER is an up-to-date source for new drug applications and for useful background information on new drugs. The medical reviews and statistician reviews can be of great value. It is worthwhile to do a search using the generic and brand names of the agents of interest at both of these sections.

The British National Health Service supports a health technology assessment program, whose purpose is to ensure that high-quality research is available on the effectiveness and cost of health technologies. This program awards funding for monographs that are produced by various people or groups who apply for grant funding. Another source to be considered is the Canadian Coordinating Office for Health Technology Assessment (CCOHTA). CCOHTA is a source for unbiased, evidence-based information on drugs, devices, health care systems, and best practices. CCOHTA is funded by Canadian federal, provincial, and territorial governments.

A few of the medical reference sources for information on clinical background and alternatives are Clinical Evidence (http://www.clinicalevidence.com), the Cochrane Collaboration (http://www.cochrane.org), Agency for Healthcare Research and Quality (http://www.ahrq.gov), DynaMed (http://www.dynamicmedical.com), and Turning Research into Practice (http://www.tripdatabase.com). However, many sources can be relied upon *only* for background information and not for drawing conclusions about efficacy because they might not be based on valid research studies. Many sources are available by subscription only; however, free access to Clinical Evidence may be obtained through the United Health Foundation (http://www.unitedhealthfoundation.org). Many times, well-done RCTs provide very helpful background information in the introduction of the article.

Ideal Study Parameters

The next step after obtaining background information is to frame a clinical question that involves consideration of the condition and the intervention. Then further background work is needed to understand potentially ideal methods for what high-quality scientific studies might look like. For example, in the ideal world, what would be the best clinical question to serve identified needs, paying particular attention to clinical significance in ways that directly benefit patients? What would the most representative patient population look like if appropriate inclusion and exclusion criteria were used? What is the ideal dosing? What might be the optimal comparison against the agent being evaluated? What are the potency equivalents for any active comparisons? What would be the ideal length of time for washout phases for various competing agents in any pretrial period or in the case of a crossover design? What would be the ideal study length? What are ideal ways to measure the outcomes?

There are several benefits for doing this preliminary background. It provides for a gold standard to which actual studies can be compared. It is also an approach that can be more instructive to reviewers, such as the typical P&T committee member who, practically speaking, will not have had the time, or often the skills, to be able to make such an assessment to evaluate the quality of the science found.

For example, if new drug, X, were being evaluated for use in atopic dermatitis, the ideal study parameters would address the following:

> ➤ The ideal study question would be directed to patient outcomes of symptom relief and improved skin appearance.
> ➤ The study design would be an RCT.
> ➤ The treatment would have a duration of 6 to 12 months.
> ➤ The new agent would be compared with the best available current care using infant, children, and adult study subjects who represent the population of interest (i.e., have appropriate inclusion and exclusion criteria such as excluding pregnant women and people taking other immunosuppressive agents).
> ➤ The dosing used would be the "usual" dosing approved by FDA.
> ➤ Clinically useful instruments for measuring improvement would be used, such as the Investigator's Global Assessment and the Eczema Area and Severity Index.
> ➤ Potency equivalents of alternative agents would be determined in advance of the review along with information on ideal washout periods.

Evidence Roundup and Assessment for Validity and Usefulness

The next step is to round up the potentially most useful evidence for assessment. The process starts with a focused clinical question to be applied for searching. Key points include using the generic and the brand name in the search because database filing might use only one name. The references in articles found in the literature search will provide keywords to help broaden the search.

Documenting the search strategy is very important. Recording the PMID number found at the bottom of each PubMed abstract can speed up retrieving a particular abstract if it is needed again. Reference managers are electronic products that assist users in locating and creating bibliographies and citation lists through automation. (Chapter 8 reviews the use of reference managers.) Including key elements from the search strategy documentation in the documents that are prepared for a drug review contributes to transparency. The following tips aid in effective filtering of information for efficiency:

1. To find the best quality information, start with trusted sources (Table 7–2) for valid, useful, and usable information. "Trusted" means that there is general agreement by EBM experts with the methods used, increasing the likelihood that the outcomes are valid. However, sometimes quality of information varies even with trusted sources; therefore, some EBM experts would advocate auditing any trusted source used and critically appraising information from all other sources.
2. Update information from trusted sources and systematic reviews, including meta-analyses:
   —Choose studies published after the source's search date, matching study type to the question (i.e., RCTs for questions of therapy, screening, and prevention).
   —Critically appraise the newer studies, especially if they are not from one of the trusted sources. (Check DARE for a critical appraisal of the article.)
3. Try the following procedure if information from a trusted source is not available:
   —Search PubMed (http://www.pubmed.org) for systematic reviews or meta-analyses: Click on the "Limits" button at the top; then from "Type of Article" select "Meta-Analysis," or from "Subsets" and "Topics" select "Systematic Reviews."
   —To specify type of article, choose "Limits" from the menu bar; then check appropriate box under "Type of Article."

Table 7–2 Trusted Sources of Clinical Evidence

Clinical Evidence (http://www.clinicalevidence.org):

➤ Evaluates and synthesizes original research
➤ Provides systematic reviews and RCTs published after the systematic reviews

The Cochrane Collaboration (http://www.cochrane.org):

➤ Evaluates and synthesizes original research
➤ Focuses on the effects of health care interventions
➤ Includes the Database of Abstracts of Reviews of Effectiveness

Database of Abstracts of Reviews of Effectiveness (DARE) (http://www.york.ac.uk/inst/crd/crddatabases. htm):

➤ Reviews potential systematic reviews, assesses them for methodologic quality against a set of inclusion criteria, and summarizes the results
➤ Flags information that is likely to be of poor quality with the words "use with caution"

Informedhealthonline (http://www.informedhealthonline.org/index.2.en.html):

➤ Provides abstracts of systematic reviews published by the Cochrane Collaboration

---

—Search PubMed for RCTs: Click on the "Limits" button at the top; then from "Publication Types" select "randomized controlled trial."
—Appraise and update articles as described earlier.
—Check out links within PubMed to comments and related articles for critical appraisal issues or something else of interest.

Searching Tips for Harms[7,8]

Large RCTs, including long-term follow-up of RCTs, should be sought, but this search is problematic if harms are rare or late:

➤ Search for systematic reviews of RCTs dealing with harms, but harms may be described in various ways in different studies.
➤ Search for case–control and cohort studies.

Appraisal for Validity and Results

Using criteria to quickly identify studies with lethal threats to validity or usability can save valuable time during critical appraisal of studies. Studies with the following characteristics usually have little clinical value:

➤ Observational studies for questions of therapy, prevention, or screening (standards may be lowered in instances of harms, but a net view should be taken).
➤ Case series (including reports using comparisons to historical controls or "natural statistics") unless all-or-none results (highly rare) are given.
➤ Results that lack clinical significance.
➤ For RCTs, study procedures or schemes that result in patients being unrandomized (e.g., exclusions postrandomization).
➤ Loss to follow-up of 5% or more without an appropriate intention-to-treat (ITT) analysis.
➤ Post hoc analyses such as those done through database research, or any research question not determined in advance.

➤ Subgroup analyses in which the subgroups were not determined in advance.

➤ Nonsignificant findings are reported; however, there were an insufficient number of patients analyzed for that outcome to show a statistically significant difference, if one existed (meaning the outcome was "underpowered"), or the number needed to reach power for that outcome is not known. (Without reaching appropriate power, it is impossible to know if no statistically significant difference truly exists or if the study population was not large enough to find a difference, provided one existed. If a statistically significant difference exists between the intervention and the comparison group, one can be certain that there was sufficient power to detect a difference.)

➤ Studies reporting intermediate markers (also known as proxy or surrogate markers), such as biologic factors (e.g., bone density) or test results (e.g., blood pressure readings) assume the intermediate markers represent a clinically meaningful outcome such as reduction in fracture or reduction in stroke. For this assumption to be valid, there must be an established, solid causal link from the intermediate marker to the clinically meaningful outcome

➤ Valid studies with clinically meaningful outcomes but for which the results are too small to be clinically helpful.

➤ Studies that are otherwise so flawed that the results cannot be trusted.

Because many authors incorrectly use various terms, the clinician must understand the concepts and not just accept what the authors say. The term *intention to treat* is often cited by authors who have not actually performed the analysis correctly. Accuracy of the analysis can be checked by evaluating whether outcomes are provided for all patients in the groups to which they were randomized and the method used for assigning outcomes for missing values.[9] The issue of loss to follow-up is frequently misunderstood. At times, loss to follow-up is greater than 5%, but the authors present an ITT analysis in which they have assigned outcomes for missing data that put the intervention through a rigorous test such as assigning positive outcomes to missing controls (i.e., assigning an outcome that all missing controls did well) and assigning negative outcomes to missing study subjects (i.e., assigning an outcome that all missing study subjects did poorly). If they have made an appropriate choice for assigning all missing outcomes, the loss to follow-up is not necessarily considered a lethal threat to validity. (Note: If the author has not performed an ITT analysis, the pharmacist may be able to perform this analysis by assigning outcomes for missing values that put the intervention or element of interest through a rigorous test.)

After first looking for these problems, the clinician should document the study reference and, if applicable, the reason for excluding a study. The list need not be complete. Any one of the above reasons can be enough to exclude a study from the review.

For studies included in an analysis, a review document with a summary of key study elements, along with a critical appraisal critique, should be prepared. This method helps provide transparency and will facilitate the discussion for formulary decision making. Each of these studies can also be graded, using one of the many grading systems for evidence review. Criteria for selecting a grading system include simplicity, ease to remember, ease to apply, comprehensibility, meaningfulness, and validity. Some systems may mix RCTs and cohort studies, for example, and give a grade of level 1 or 2 for these studies. These grades can make the evidence sound better than it actually is because only valid RCTs with usable results should be applied to address questions of therapy.

Summarize and Synthesize the Evidence

The goal of evidence synthesis is to take all of the best available valid and useful evidence one has found and summarize it into a conclusion. The evidence synthesis is usually a text statement in which one makes claims from the evidence. This step generally entails applying a great deal of judgment. Language that is inaccurate, misleading, or vague, such as "the evidence suggests...," or "it is likely to be shown that...," or "there is some evidence that..." should be avoided.

As with individual studies reviewed, applying a grade to evidence synthesis is recommended. The grade applies to the strength of the evidence found. For example, evidence to be summarized may be moderate or weak; the grade applied to the synthesis should reflect that. Finally, a statement of any limitations of the review and the subsequent synthesis should accompany the synthesis.

A conservative approach is recommended for the following reasons:

1. Study biases frequently favor the intervention (and all studies have some bias).
2. Long-term harms may not show up for an extended period of time—and are infrequently found in the initial research.
3. The results of research within a research setting (efficacy) are usually better than the results seen in clinical practice (effectiveness).

The following statement is a hypothetical example of an evidence synthesis statement; Table 7-3 presents the generic format:

> Grade A Evidence: There is strong evidence of efficacy favoring drug X. It can be concluded that there is benefit in reducing hip and other fractures for high-risk females older than 65 years at risk when taking drug X compared with placebo within 3 years. The ARR for 3 years is 4% (95% CI, 2%–5%). NNT for clinically meaningful improvement in reduction of risk for fracture is estimated at NNT of 20–50 (3 years). Harms and potential harms include 2% chance of stomach upset and 0.5% of gastric ulcer, and may include other risks as longer-term data become available. NNH is estimated at NNH of 50–200 (3 years).

Table 7-3 Format Example for Evidence Synthesis Statements

[Grade A: Strong; Grade B: Potentially Strong] Evidence: There is [Strong; Potentially Strong] evidence of efficacy. It can be concluded that there is benefit in [clinically significant area] for [patients] with [condition] [population inclusions/exclusions] taking [agent] when compared with [comparator] within [study duration] as measured with [measurement instrument]. The ARR for [study period] is [ARR%] (95% CI, [CI–CI%]. NNT for clinically meaningful [improvement] in [clinically significant area] is estimated at NNT of [CI] [(study duration)]. Harms and potential harms include [list statistically significant harms and quantify; add other harms as seems appropriate] and may include other risks as longer-term data become available. NNH is estimated at NNH of [CI] [(study duration)]. Potential harms data [are/are not] from an RCT. Harms data [are/are not] from case reports or case series. Study [was/was not] powered for harms. Or—

[Grade U Evidence: There is uncertain evidence of efficacy due to [list issues with challenges to validity and/or lack of clinical usefulness]. [Harms information may be described as noted above.]

ARR = Absolute risk reduction; NNT = number needed to treat; NNH = number needed to harm; RCT = randomized controlled trial.

Project Potential Impacts of Practice Change

As stated earlier, a truly evidence- and value-based process considers impacts of practice change, taking the net view into account. In many instances, practice change impacts can be assessed by looking at the current processes of care and related considerations, and comparing them to imagined possible resulting changes. This assessment entails consideration of impacts on the patient and physician perspective; satisfaction for patients and providers; impacts of utilization, such as effects on facilities, systems, roles and skills needed, methods, procedures, equipment, supplies and other resources, and on the other triangulation issues; and, importantly, cost.

For example, when considering the addition of an immunomodulating drug for atopic dermatitis, one would want to consider not only the efficacy, but estimates of change in office visits, utilization of corticosteroids, referrals to specialists and utilization of other immunomodulating drugs, patient and clinician satisfaction, and cost.

Cost assessment is an area that is frequently a key responsibility for P&T committees—and, therefore, clinical pharmacist staff supporting those committees. Frequently those involved in determining methods for doing a cost review will choose from a wide array of potentially confusing methods. The best method is choosing a method that is appropriate to the need, but which is the most simple and comprehensible of the appropriate choices. Frequently, for most health care organizations, a simple cost-analysis approach, applying the average wholesale price may be adequate. Also, sometimes a simple before-and-after comparison is sufficient without trying to make the analysis too laborious. It is often enough to have an estimate of how much care will be improved and costs reduced without necessarily carrying out cost-effectiveness or cost-utility analyses.

The best approach for cost assessments is to break down all assumptions and costs into base unit values to attain transparency and greater flexibility.

An efficient and effective way to compare multiple agents is to use number needed to treat (NNT). A vitally important, and often overlooked, consideration for using NNT is the time period associated with NNT (which is the same as the study time period). Consideration of the time period is just as important as the number of people needed to treat when considering efficacy. For example, an NNT of three that can be expected to benefit patients within 1 year is potentially more effective than an NNT of three that can be expected to benefit patients within 5 years. Average cost-effectiveness analysis asks the question: What am I spending for each outcome gained? Ascertaining the cost-per-benefit can be very helpful. One needs three variables: the NNT, the study time period, and the cost for a single study time period unit, such as 1 year if the study time period is expressed as years.

Sometimes the answer will be very clear. In the example in Table 7–4, drug Y emerges as the best choice provided the clinician has examined all other factors, such as validity of studies, usefulness of results, safety considerations, application issues, and other triangulation issues, as described earlier in this chapter.

In other instances, the choice may not be immediately clear because of complexities arising from variations within the combination of NNT, time period, and/or cost. For example, which of the following agents in Table 7–5 appears to be the better agent?

When these kinds of combinations occur, a simple calculation provides useful information: NNT × study time period × cost per study time period unit. Using the example in Table 7–5, one can compute the cost-per-benefit of drug X to be $2000 and the cost-per-benefit of drug Y to be $1800. If one assumes that the research behind each agent is valid and clinically useful, and that there are no other critical differences in terms of harms, drug administration, and

Table 7–4   Agents With Variable NNTs and Time Periods but Same 1-Year Cost

Agent	NNT	Time Period	Cost for 1 Year of Treatment
Drug X	3	1 year	$100 per year
Drug Y	3	5 years	$100 per year

NNT = Number needed to treat.

Table 7–5   Agents With Variable Treatment Periods, NNTs, and 1-Year Costs

Agent	NNT	Time Period	Cost for 1 Year of Treatment
Drug X	5	4 years	$100 per year
Drug Y	4	5 years	$90 per year

NNT = Number needed to treat.

Table 7–6   Average Cost-Effectiveness Analysis

Agent	NNT	Time Period	Cost for 1 Year of Treatment	Cost-per-Benefit
Drug X	5	4 years	$100 per year	$5 \times 4 \times 100 = \$2000$
Drug Y	4	5 years	$90 per year	$4 \times 5 \times \ 90 = \$1800$

NNT = Number needed to treat.

so forth, this calculation is a simple way to compute an average cost-effectiveness analysis (as shown in Table 7–6), which can yield helpful information to achieve greater value.

Various scenarios might be worthwhile to consider. Some useful ways to view the data would be to do a best-case and a worst-case scenario, to consider confidence intervals, and to assess estimates for effectiveness compared with efficacy. An online calculator, available at http://www.delfini.org, can help in computing these comparative calculations.

About Pharmacoeconomic Studies

Many groups use pharmacoeconomic studies to help them with economic analysis. Such a study may be available in PubMed. However, all pharmacoeconomic studies, unless they are from one of the trusted sources in Table 7–2, need to be critically appraised for validity and usefulness (and it is advisable to audit even those from a trusted source). The following additional considerations for quality and applicable pharmacoeconomic studies also need to be addressed.

Pharmacoeconomic analysis essentially entails combining several elements into an economic model, meaning that a construct is created in an attempt to help predict what may happen in clinical practice. The elements that create the model include health care outcomes, which should be based on valid and useful RCTs, cost data and assumptions such as the number of patients projected to make an office visit, estimated number of patients who will be prescribed a particular medication or projected number of patients who will experience an adverse event, and so on.

The first and foremost consideration is to determine whether and how the authors critically appraised the studies included in the model. Often, this important step is neglected in pharmacoeconomic studies. Second, evidence is usually a global consideration, while cost is a local one. Cost outcomes published in a national journal article—and based on a national perspective—may not have relevance for the group using the data. Third, assumptions are assumptions. Even when based on data, assumptions are opinions, estimates, conjectures, or guesses—and like cost—assumptions are likely to be local. A practitioner's assumptions, based on local considerations, may be as meaningful or more meaningful than those used in a study. A practitioner may find it worthwhile to create a model based on local considerations and then use pharmacoeconomic studies for ideas or inputs to create and adjust the model.

It may be best to obtain and use a tool that is appropriate for evaluating pharmacoeconomic studies before using the studies. (Appendix 6–A in Chapter 6 provides aids for evaluating these studies: Web tutorials, sample scenarios, and an appraisal worksheet.) Practitioners might want to consider the following criteria, at a minimum, to determine the appropriateness of a study for their practice:

- ➤ Did the authors critically appraise any studies on which they based their effectiveness projections for health care outcomes, and did they use only valid and clinically useful studies?
- ➤ Is the information relevant to the practitioner's circumstances?
- ➤ Is the mode of economic analysis appropriate for the local practice?
- ➤ Is the best information or reasonable assumptions included in the model?
- ➤ Were reasonable alternatives compared?
- ➤ Were sensitivity analyses conducted to test various scenarios (e.g., worst case, efficacy versus effectiveness)?
- ➤ Do limitations and biases exist?

Summarize Drug Review and Make Recommendations

The final step in conducting the drug review is to create a concluding summary. This summary should be the "roll up" for all the preceding information that has been reviewed and synthesized. The summary should be very clear and transparent about what is evidence and what is a judgment. It should address findings on evidence and safety, appropriate patient population, value assessment, comparison to alternatives, implications of practice change, and recommendations. There should be an attempt to assess the possible physician perspective (e.g., satisfaction, acceptability, likelihood of appropriate application, and actionability) and the patient perspective (e.g., benefits, costs, risks, harms, uncertainties, and alternatives), along with issues that may affect patient adherence to treatment, dependency or abuse potential, and so on. The summary should also describe limitations of the overall review and analysis. Finally, many clinical pharmacists are expected to consult with clinicians and others to make recommendations for committee consideration (including guidance, restrictions, and exclusions, consideration of substitutions, prior authorizations, and overrides).

Conclusion

This detailed model is presented to help practitioners create an effective drug review system that will inform formulary decision making. This approach includes details about how to find and critically appraise the best medical evidence, how to determine value, how to perform an economic drug review, and how to effectively—and efficiently—use the results to ensure high quality of the information that is used to support formulary decisions. In essence, this model considers the weight of the scientific evidence, the net benefits and harms, costs, and other triangulation issues required to inform decision makers about a new agent: Is its clinical value superior to, equal to, or lesser than existing agents?

The Bottom Line

The steps to an explicit evidence-based formulary are referred to as the "five A's" of EBM:

➤ Ask where significant gaps within the formulary exist.
➤ Acquire information using evidence-based techniques, which include a systematic search and appropriate filtering techniques.
➤ Appraise information for validity, usefulness, and value.
➤ Apply information by careful crafting of conclusions to create information, decision, and action aids, and by implementing new therapy programs, measuring the success of implementation and performance, and reporting key outcomes.
➤ Again, cycle back through preceding steps to continuously improve clinical care.

Transparency through good documentation of all steps and reporting is critical to good evidence-based practice.

References

1. Centers for Medicare and Medicaid Services. Health care spending in the United States slows for the first time in seven years [news release]. Tuesday, January 11, 2005. Available at: http://www.cms.hhs.gov/media/press/release.asp?Counter=1314. Accessed October 23, 2006.

2. Chassin MR, Galvin RW, and the National Roundtable on Health Care Quality. The urgent need to improve health care quality. *JAMA.* 1998;280:1000–5.

3. McGlynn EA, Asch SM, Adams J, et al. The quality of health care delivered to adults in the United States. *N Engl J Med.* 2003;348:2635–45.

4. Kerr EA, McGlynn EA, Adams J. Profiling the quality of care in twelve communities: results from the CQI study. *Health Affairs.* 2004;23(3):247–56.

5. Stergachis A. Pharmacoeconomics [PowerPoint presentation]. Presented at the King County Healthcare Advisory Task Force Meeting, March 8, 2004, Seattle, Washington.

6. Eddy DM. Clinical decision making: from theory to practice. The challenge. *JAMA.* 1990;263(2):287–90.

7. Vandenbroucke JP. Benefits and harms of drug treatments. *BMJ.* 2004;329(7456):2–3. PMID: 15231587.

8. Greenhalgh T, Kostopoulou O, Harries C. Making decisions about benefits and harms of medicines. *BMJ.* 2004;329(7456):47–50. PMID: 15231628.

9. Pitkin RM, Branagan MA, Burmeister LF. Accuracy of data in abstracts of published research articles. *JAMA.* 1999; 281:1110–1.

APPENDIX 7–A
GLOSSARY OF DRUG REVIEW TERMS

Class effect: The state of agents having clinical effects considered sufficiently similar (i.e., equipotency) to allow grouping them into one drug family or "drug class." (For all intents and purposes, class effect treats the agents as if they are the same clinically, but some other factors, such as cost, may vary.)

Drug utilization review (DUR): A system for evaluating appropriateness of drug therapy. Prescribing patterns are evaluated to determine if drugs are being misprescribed, possibly resulting in problems with safety or effectiveness.

Equipotency: The state of agents having clinical effects considered sufficiently similar (i.e., class effect) to allow grouping them into one drug family or "drug class." (For all intents and purposes, equipotency treats the agents as if they are the same clinically, but some other factors, such as cost, may vary.)

First-line therapy: The drugs to be utilized first in treating a patient.

Formulary: List of therapeutic agents available in a particular practice for caring for patients. The term "preferred drug list" is also used.

> ➤ An open formulary may have few or no restrictions.
> ➤ A closed formulary has restrictions.

Formulary system: A system that provides for the processes for establishing and managing the formulary.

Generic substitution: Replacement of one agent with a different agent having the same chemical structure, which may occur when the patent on a brand-name drug expires. Bioequivalence is frequently assumed (i.e., it is assumed that the generic agent is equivalent to the brand-name drug). In some cases the effects of other components of the generic preparation (e.g., the vehicle in a dermatologic preparation) may vary and result in outcomes that differ from those reported for the brand-name agent.

Monograph: A written review and analysis, often of a single agent, containing a list of usage recommendations.

Narrative review: An article in the medical literature summarizing other studies for a given topic, characterized by a lack of a transparent, scientific, and systematic approach; thus, the summary is highly likely to be misleading. Instead, systematic reviews should be sought (and appraised).

Override: Process of setting aside a prescriber's choice of a medication and usually substituting another medication.

Pharmacy & Therapeutics (P&T) Committee: Committee charged with making formulary management decisions, along with performing other formulary management functions.

Pharmacy benefit manager (PBM): A company that manages pharmacy benefits and formulary management for health care systems and/or insurance companies.

Prior authorization: Requirement that a clinician obtain approval before a drug can be dispensed and/or covered.

Rebate: A cost offset that pharmacy systems receive when purchasing large quantities of drugs.

Second-line therapy: Therapy for patients failing on drugs established as "first-line" therapy.

Systematic review: An article in the medical literature summarizing other studies for a given topic, using a transparent, scientific, and systematic approach to identify and include valid and useful studies in the review. A meta-analysis is a subset of systematic reviews, characterized by how the results of the studies are combined quantitatively and statistically. Unless retrieved from trusted sources, systematic reviews need to be critically appraised for validity and usability. (It is advisable to audit trusted sources for validity and clinical usefulness.)

Therapeutic substitution: Substitution of a drug with an agent having a different chemical structure but similar clinical benefits.

Triangulation issues: A catchall term for all the various considerations that need to be made in making a decision.

KEEPING UP TO DATE

L. Michael Posey and Elaine Chiquette

$\mathcal{M}$OST OF THE SITUATIONS DESCRIBED thus far in *Evidence-Based Pharmacotherapy* presume that a unique question or situation has been presented to the clinician and that a literature search will provide evidence that can be used to develop a rational therapeutic approach. However, most clinicians—including pharmacists—have a standard approach to management of the more commonly seen conditions in their practices. An ongoing need for these clinicians is to know when to revise their usual patterns on the basis of research being presented at medical meetings and published in journals.

The task sounds simpler than it is. We live in an information society in which knowledge doubles every few years and patients hear about the latest clinical research on television or read about it on the Internet before most clinicians get off work. How then does one keep up to date on advances in clinical research, new drug approvals, and emerging safety concerns, and use that information to update treatment paradigms in daily practice?

Clinical Research: Sorting Out the Cacophony of Evidence

The task of staying current is a formidable one. The National Library of Medicine, through *Index Medicus,* MEDLINE, and PubMed, covers nearly 4800 journals and contains more than 13 million bibliographic citations, as of November 2006.[1] Results of more than 10,000 randomized controlled trials are published each year, along with thousands of meta-analyses and systematic reviews. With the many other types of studies and reports in journals, clinicians cannot humanly keep track of every possible publication that might affect their practices. As described in Chapter 2, finding just the right study can truly be like looking for a needle in a haystack.

Despite this challenge, clinicians can keep up with relevant literature and advances in the therapeutic areas important in their practices. Doing so is a matter of simply following the same procedure used to resolve patient-specific pharmacotherapeutic questions: (1) recognize one's information needs, (2) identify literature relevant to those needs, (3) critically appraise the evidence for validity and utility, and (4) devise a mechanism to incorporate new evidence into daily practice.

From among the tens of thousands of journals (not all are included in MEDLINE), pharmacists need to determine which are so important to their practices that they must be received and read (or at least scanned) each month. For generalist pharmacists, the choice may be the pharmacy journals relevant to their practice setting, along with perhaps an internal medicine journal or general medical publication. For pharmacists specializing in certain therapeutic areas, journals in those organ systems or disease states—especially those publications with gold standard randomized controlled trials—will be important (Table 8–1).

When reviewing the journals of interest is not possible, health professionals can subscribe to literature monitoring or retrieval services, such as those listed in Table 8–2. These services, which offer Web-based information, push e-mail messages, and print documents, can greatly reduce the time needed to monitor the literature, assuming that the scope of their monitoring closely matches the practitioner's areas of practice.

Table 8–1   Key Journals in Selected Therapeutic Areas

Therapeutic Areas	Key Journals	Web Sites
General medicine	*The New England Journal of Medicine*	http://content.nejm.org
	JAMA (Journal of the American Medical Association)	http://www.jama.com
	Lancet	http://www.thelancet.com
	BMJ (formerly the *British Medical Journal)*	http://www.bmj.org
General clinical research and pharmacy practice	*Pharmacotherapy*	http://www.pharmacotherapy.org
	Journal of the American Pharmacists Association	http://www.japha.org
	American Journal of Health-System Pharmacy	http://www.ashp.org/ajhp/index.cfm
	Annals of Pharmacotherapy	http://www.amcp.org
Internal medicine	*Annals of Internal Medicine*	http://www.theannals.com
	Archives of Internal Medicine	http://www.archinternalmed.com
Cardiology	*Journal of the American College of Cardiology*	http://www.cardiosource.com
	Circulation	http://circ.ahajournals.org
Pulmonology	*Chest*	http://www.chestnet.org
	American Journal of Respiratory and Critical Care Medicine	http://ajrccm.atsjournals.org
Gastroenterology	*Gastroenterology*	http://www.gastrojournal.org
Nephrology	*American Journal of Kidney Diseases*	http://www.ajkd.org
Neurology	*Neurology*	http://www.neurology.org
	Archives of Neurology	http://www.archneurol.com
Psychiatry	*American Journal of Psychiatry*	http://www.ajp.psychiatryonline.org
	Archives of General Psychiatry	http://www.archgenpsychiatry.com
Endocrinology	*Diabetes Care*	http://care.diabetesjournals.org
	Obesity	http://www.obesityresearch.org
Urology	*Journal of Urology*	http://www.jurology.com
Immunology	*Journal of Allergy and Clinical Immunology*	http://www.jacionline.org
Rheumatology	*Arthritis & Rheumatism*	http://www.rheumatology.org/publications/index.asp

Table 8–1 (continued) Key Journals in Selected Therapeutic Areas

Therapeutic Areas	Key Journals	Web Sites
Otolaryngology	*Archives of Otolaryngology*	http://archotol.ama-assn.org
Dermatology	*Archives of Dermatology*	http://archderm.ama-assn.org
Hematology/ oncology	*Cancer*	http://www3.interscience.wiley.com/ cgi-bin/jhome/28741
	Journal of Clinical Oncology	http://www.jco.org
Infectious diseases	*Clinical Infectious Diseases*	http://www.journals.uchicago.edu/ CID/home.html
	Antimicrobial Agents and Chemotherapy	http://aac.asm.org
	Journal of Acquired Immune Deficiency Syndromes	http://www.jaids.com
Nutrition	*Journal of Parenteral and Enteral Nutrition*	http://jpen.aspenjournals.org/
Pediatrics	*Pediatrics*	http://www.pediatrics.org
	The Journal of Pediatrics	http://journals.elsevierhealth.com/ periodicals/ympd
Geriatrics	*Journal of the American Geriatrics Society*	http://www.blackwell-synergy.com
Other	*Health Affairs*	http://www.healthaffairs.org
	Medical Care	http://www.lww-medicalcare.com

Table 8–2 Services for Keeping Up With the Biomedical Literature

Service/(Web Site)/Purpose	Audience	Selection Criteria	No. of Journals Scanned/Scope of Literature Coverage
ACP Journal Club (http://www.acpjc.org/?hp) "To select from the biomedical literature articles that report original studies and systematic reviews that warrant immediate attention by physicians attempting to keep pace with important advances in internal medicine"	Internal medicine, primary care	Articles must be in English, be about adult humans, be about topics (other than descriptive studies of prevalence) that are important to general internal medicine and analyze data consistently with the study question	>100
Bandolier (http://www.jr2.ox.ac.uk/ bandolier) "Evidence based thinking about health care"	Various	Publishes an 8-page monthly journal and books; also offers individualized training courses; is active in the areas of pain and pain research	Monthly searches of PubMed and the Cochrane Library for recent systematic reviews and meta-analyses

Table 8–2 (continued)   Services for Keeping Up With the Biomedical Literature

Service/(Web Site)/Purpose	Audience	Selection Criteria	No. of Journals Scanned/Scope of Literature Coverage
Clinical Evidence (http://www.clinicalevidence.org/ceweb/conditions/index.jsp) Promotes informed decision making by summarizing "what's known—and not known—about more than 200 medical conditions and over 2000 treatments"	Primary and hospital care	Studies of sufficient quality are used to formulate evidence on treatment of medical conditions; process is repeated for each topic every 12 months to incorporate new studies	Main sources: Cochrane databases, MEDLINE, Embase, and other databases as appropriate
Evidence-Based Mental Health (http://ebmh.bmjjournals.com) Alerts clinicians to important advances in treatment, diagnosis, etiology, prognosis, continuing education, economic evaluation, and qualitative research in mental health	Clinicians	Applies strict criteria for the quality and validity of research and obtains assessment of clinical relevance by practicing clinicians; presents results in succinct, informative abstract with expert commentary	"Wide range of international medical journals"
Journal Watch Online (http://www.jwatch.org) Physician-authored summaries and commentary from the publishers of the *New England Journal of Medicine*	Physicians and other health professionals	Physician editors systematically review and filter journals, and supply concise summaries and insightful commentary	More than 180 medical and scientific journals
PNN Pharmacotherapy News Network (http://homepage.mac.com/lmposey/PNN/index.html) Provides news and information about medications and their proper use	Pharmacists	Daily e-mail newsletter covering important new studies in journals and at medical meetings, FDA actions, and related news events	Major medical weeklies; internal medicine journals; top 1 or 2 journals in most clinical areas; pharmacy journals

Many of these services, in addition to alerting subscribers to new articles, also critically appraise studies and provide evidence ratings or commentaries about them. This information further assists practitioners as they seek to determine the clinical relevance of data reported in clinical trials.

As new information emerges and is analyzed, the individual practitioner must then decide whether to change the way diseases are treated in individual patients. As this happens, the evidence-based pharmacotherapy steps are completed, and the practitioner continues to monitor the literature for important new evidence that will further improve patient care.

Bibliographic Management Software

Many practitioners have an electronic library organized with folders, but still cannot find an article read a month ago. Or organizing the references for an article to be published is a nightmare (not the right citation format for the journal or hours must be spent typing the citations). A bibliographic management software program will help manage citations retrieved from a wide variety of formats (Internet, PubMed, Ovid, Current Contents, etc.). This type of software is a powerful tool providing flexible organization and manipulation of references. It is referred to by many names, including citation management software, personal bibliographic managers, reference managers, information management tools, bibliographic software, but all the programs perform the same functions.

This software is now so common that most medical journals offer to download articles directly to a reference/citation manager (Figure 8–1). Some examples of how the software can help practitioners manage their library of articles, slides, Web sites, and so on are illustrated in the following scenario and other discussions.

∽
Scenario
∽

You are completing a search on Ovid for a review article you are writing. There are several references that you will pull and most likely include as references in the manuscript. Luckily you have a reference manager software on your computer, allowing you to download the citations directly from Ovid. You are using Microsoft Word as your word processor. Because your reference manager is compatible with Microsoft Word, you can "cite as you write," meaning that your Word document is directly linked to your reference manager software and citations are added in the correct order and in the desired format as you write the review article.

Reference managers can convert and import bibliographic data (citation and the full abstract if available) from external electronic sources such as Ovid, PubMed, medical journals, or Web sites. The software also allows the user to search PubMed or other electronic databases directly within the software. For example, in the keeping-up-to-date mode, one can import the citations of interest from a monthly search to the reference manager. Or if one finds an article of interest during a browse of a monthly journal, it is very likely that the journal offers a direct download of the citation to a reference manager (Figure 8–1). Furthermore, if a PDF of the article is downloaded, the PDF can be linked to the citation in the reference manager, allowing the reference manager to be opened later and the search engine used to retrieve not only the citation but also the PDF.

Once a database is created for a specific project, citations can be further classified into categories (categories can be thought of as folders), or new searchable keywords added. The entire database can be searched for a text word within the title or abstract. The search engine within the reference manager software is fairly sophisticated and will allow advanced search strategies with Boolean terms.

The software allows creation of bibliographies with selected or all citations formatted for either the *New England Journal of Medicine*, or *JAMA*, or *Archives of Internal Medicine*, or for a customized output format. The citations can be exported directly into a Word document to facilitate the task of creating a bibliography for a manuscript.

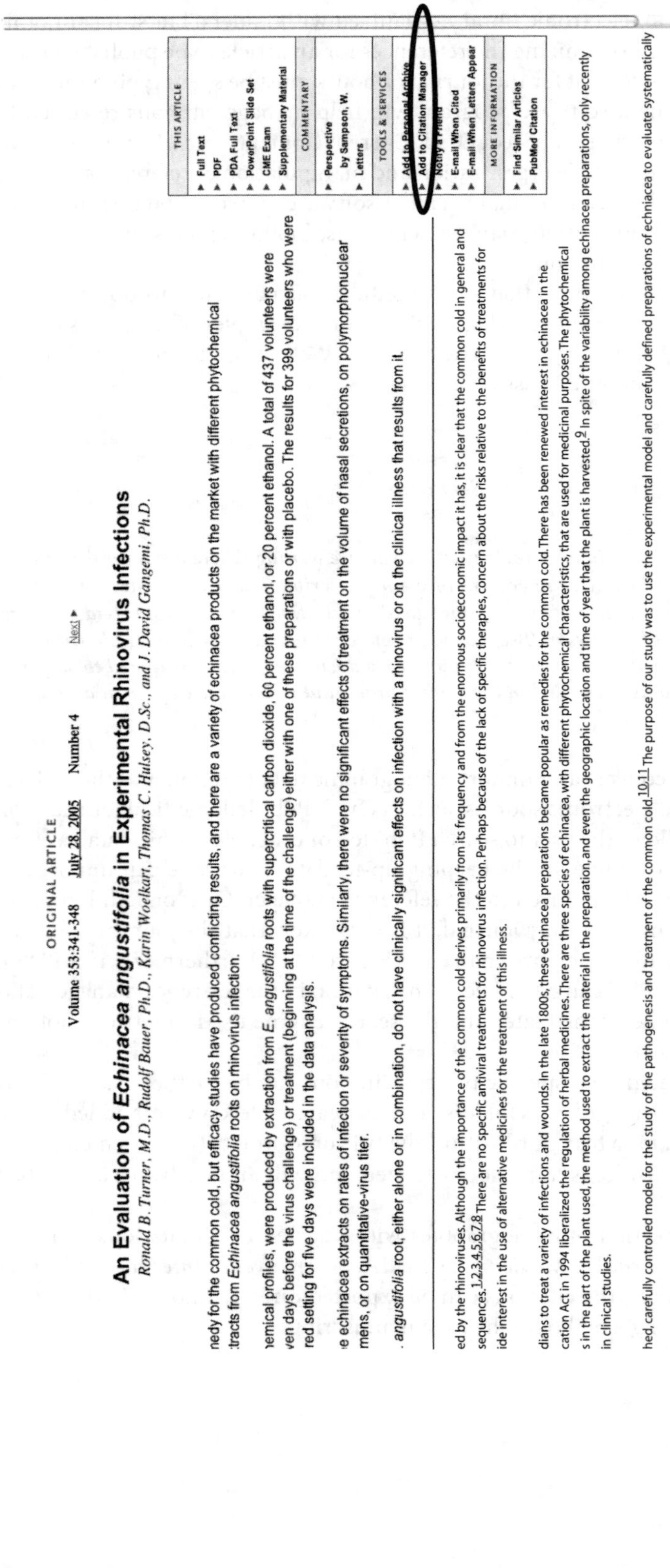
ORIGINAL ARTICLE
Volume 353:341-348 July 28, 2005 Number 4 Next ▸
An Evaluation of Echinacea angustifolia in Experimental Rhinovirus Infections
Ronald B. Turner, M.D., Rudolf Bauer, Ph.D., Karin Woelkart, Thomas C. Hulsey, D.Sc., and J. David Gangemi, Ph.D.
nedy for the common cold, but efficacy studies have produced conflicting results, and there are a variety of echinacea products on the market with different phytochemical
tracts from Echinacea angustifolia roots on rhinovirus infection.
nemical profiles, were produced by extraction from E. angustifolia roots with supercritical carbon dioxide, 60 percent ethanol, or 20 percent ethanol. A total of 437 volunteers were
ven days before the virus challenge) or treatment (beginning at the time of the challenge) either with one of these preparations or with placebo. The results for 399 volunteers who were
red setting for five days were included in the data analysis.
e echinacea extracts on rates of infection or severity of symptoms. Similarly, there were no significant effects of treatment on the volume of nasal secretions, on polymorphonuclear
mens, or on quantitative-virus titer.
. angustifolia root, either alone or in combination, do not have clinically significant effects on infection with a rhinovirus or on the clinical illness that results from it.
ed by the rhinoviruses. Although the importance of the common cold derives primarily from its frequency and from the enormous socioeconomic impact it has, it is clear that the common cold in general and
sequences.1,2,3,4,5,6,7,8 There are no specific antiviral treatments for rhinovirus infection. Perhaps because of the lack of specific therapies, concern about the risks relative to the benefits of treatments for
ide interest in the use of alternative medicines for the treatment of this illness.
dians to treat a variety of infections and wounds. In the late 1800s, these echinacea preparations became popular as remedies for the common cold. There has been renewed interest in echinacea in the
cation Act in 1994 liberalized the regulation of herbal medicines. There are three species of echinacea, with different phytochemical characteristics, that are used for medicinal purposes. The phytochemical
s in the part of the plant used, the method used to extract the material in the preparation, and even the geographic location and time of year that the plant is harvested.9 In spite of the variability among echinacea preparations, only recently
in clinical studies.
hed, carefully controlled model for the study of the pathogenesis and treatment of the common cold.10,11 The purpose of our study was to use the experimental model and carefully defined preparations of echinacea to evaluate systematically
THIS ARTICLE
▸ Full Text
▸ PDF
▸ PDA Full Text
▸ PowerPoint Slide Set
▸ CME Exam
▸ Supplementary Material
COMMENTARY
▸ Perspective by Sampson, W.
▸ Letters
TOOLS & SERVICES
▸ Add to Personal Archive
▸ Add to Citation Manager
▸ Notify a Friend
▸ E-mail When Cited
▸ E-mail When Letters Appear
MORE INFORMATION
▸ Find Similar Articles
▸ PubMed Citation

Figure 8–1

Downloading articles directly from a journal's Web site to a reference manager. *The New England Journal of Medicine* as well as several other medical journals offer the option to download the citation directly to a reference/citation/bibliographic manager.

Table 8–3   Comparison of Bibliographic Management Software

Feature	ProCite	Reference Manager	EndNote
Search the Internet	Yes	Yes	Yes
Store and cite images	No	No	Yes
Number of fields	45	37	52
Subject bibliography	Yes	Yes	Yes
Format bibliographies	Yes	Yes	Yes
Advance searching	Yes	No	No
Cite while you write	Yes	Yes	Yes
Link to PDF on the Internet or desktop	Yes	Yes	Yes
Access open URL link	Yes	Yes	Yes

The three most commonly used bibliographic management programs are EndNote, Pro-Cite, and Reference Manager, which are all produced by Thomson ISI ResearchSoft. Table 8–3 describes the strengths and weaknesses of each program. The CD-ROM included with this book includes an executable demo and tutorial for ProCite, and provides information about free trial demos and online tutorials for the other two programs.

PEACEFUL: Getting the Most from Pharmaceutical Industry Field Representative Visits

The pharmaceutical industry is also a good source of information. When drugs are first marketed, it is often the only source of information for the drugs. Thus, while clinicians must assess possible bias in communications, they also must learn to get the information they need from the companies that market medications.

A primary means of communications to most clinicians is through the pharmaceutical industry field representative; this process, called drug detailing, can be an effective way for pharmacists to gain up-to-date information about new drugs. Drug detailing is a one-on-one meeting in which pharmaceutical representatives present information included in their product's label. Academic detailing is a one-on-one meeting in which a trained health care professional (not affiliated with an organization for profit) educates the physician on a new intervention or drug. The value of drug detailing is controversial. The criticism has been that the information provided from pharmaceutical representatives is biased, inaccurate, and oftentimes irrelevant. The key for successful interaction with pharmaceutical field representatives is to take charge of the interview, set the agenda, ask for references, and apply the evidence-based pharmacotherapy principles to the data provided by the drug representative. Shaughnessy and his colleagues created the acronym STEPS—safety, tolerability, effectiveness, price, and simplicity—to help frame the information needs during a visit with a field representative. Various topics are available on the STEPS page on the American Academy of Family Physicians Web site (http://www.aafp.org/afp/accessories/browse/?op=get_documents_via_department_id&department_id=12).

The acronym PEACEFUL can help the practitioner remember the elements of a focused, comprehensive, and valuable interaction with the field representative:

P = Patient's profile best suited for the new drug
E = Efficacy of the new drug compared with placebo and gold standard
A = Availability on hospital or health plan formularies
C = Cost
E = Ease of use/convenience
F = Formulations (e.g., tablets, capsules, injections, syrups)
U = Unwanted side effects (minor and major)
L = Lay educational material (video, pamphlets)

One approach is to ask the field representatives to fill out the "PEACEFUL" tool in Appendix 8–A of this chapter and to support the statements with peer-reviewed published evidence, where applicable, before the scheduled meeting. Scheduled meetings best maximize the interaction and manage the practitioner's time. For a new product, 15 to 30 minutes give ample time to review the PEACEFUL tool and assess the evidence brought by the field representative. This strategy will ensure a focused meeting targeting the discussion to the practitioner's information needs. The "leave behinds" should be only the published literature requested by the practitioner, who should beware of marketing visual aids referencing "unpublished data on file."

Patient's Profile

What is the Food and Drug Administration (FDA)-approved indication for this new drug? Who should receive it? Who should not receive it? The discussion should focus on the demographics of the subjects included and excluded from the pivotal trials conducted to achieve FDA approval for the specific indication. The field representative is restricted to a discussion on the FDA-approved labeling for the drug, but the practitioner should examine the pivotal clinical trials' Methods section and the demographic tables to get a better sense of the population studied with the drug. For example, the drug is approved for combination therapy with metformin (various manufacturers) for patients with type 2 diabetes; however, after looking at the demographic table of the pivotal trials, it is clear that the drug was given to patients with early disease (less than 4 years since diabetes was diagnosed and A1c of less than 8.5%) and that all subjects on drug Y were excluded because of possible drug interactions.

The practitioner should find out which types of patients have not been studied (most likely pregnant women, children, patients with major concomitant diseases such as liver, heart, or renal disease) or clearly should not receive the drug (because of drug interactions or concomitant disease).

Efficacy

The best efficacy data will be supported by more than one randomized controlled trial for comparing clinical outcomes of the new drug against the drug in a formulary. However, a direct comparison is most likely not available. Often the industry will sponsor head-to-head comparisons on questionable surrogate markers (in vitro type data, cellular receptors binding, etc.) and claim superiority over the competitor. In a keeping-up-to-date mode, time should not be lost discussing esoteric evidence that may or may not be relevant to clinical practice in the next decade; Patient-Oriented Evidence that Matters (POEMs) should be the focus. More likely, the new drug will be superior to placebo (because it received FDA approval), and few data comparing the new drug to the current gold standard will be available. The following points should be the focus of the meeting:

> Accept only a high level of evidence for therapeutic interventions (i.e., systematic reviews/meta-analysis or randomized controlled trials) published in independent peer-reviewed journals (not company-sponsored symposia).

> Do not be deceived by statements of relative risk reductions; instead calculate the absolute risk reductions (see Chapter 5) and respective numbers needed to treat.

> Bottom line: Observe the principles of critical appraisal for all published literature provided by the field representative.

> Avoid a discussion about the glossy marketing handout; the discussion should be about requested literature that supports the efficacy and safety of the drug for the approved indication.

Availability

Is the new drug reimbursed by Medicare/Medicaid or by the most common health plans in a particular practice? Is it on the hospital formulary? Have other institutions included the new drug in their disease management pathways?

Cost

The indirect costs should also be considered in the cost comparison with the current favorite. For example, the new drug may require extra pharmacist time to prepare or extra physician visits to monitor for possible serious adverse effects. The packaging may not be compatible with PIXIS (a medication delivery device) and similar equipment, leading to additional costs for extra staff time to get the product to the floor.

Ease of Use

The new drug may be no better than the current formulary alternative, but might offer a convenience advantage that translates to lower indirect cost (e.g., the new drug does not require the pharmacist to premix or does not require extra laboratory monitoring) or better adherence and acceptance by patients (e.g., a once-a-day dose versus four times a day, no need to refrigerate, or no drug interaction with common nonprescription drugs).

Formulations

The field representative should be asked about the formulations available for the new drug: Is it available as a syrup, suppository, injection, or patch? What are the needs of particular patients or facility vis-á-vis the available formulations?

Unwanted Effects

This information is omitted most often by the field representative. Discussion of safety with the field representative should cover the serious adverse events and the less serious but most common adverse events. Serious, possibly life-threatening adverse effects should be examined to determine whether the drug would require additional medical supervision (visits or laboratory tests) and whether its risks outweigh the superior efficacy. "How does it compare to the current gold standard?" is another important comparison. The longer a drug is on the market, the greater is the number of individuals who have been exposed to it, and the greater are the chances that more risks have been identified. The serious adverse events are often rare and may or may not be discovered in pivotal trials of short duration that expose relatively small numbers of patients (e.g., less than 3000 patients) to the new drug.

In addition, the practitioner will want to examine the most common adverse events reported in the pivotal trials because these events should likely be part of the patient counseling for this new drug. Identifying the percentage of patients who dropped out of the trial because of adverse events will determine how severe and bothersome the adverse events are.

Lay Educational Material

Pharmaceutical companies often offer excellent patient tools to facilitate patient counseling. The tools provide patient-friendly information on the disease, and/or the risks and benefits of the new drug. The format can vary from videos, brochures, and Web sites to a hotline supported by a health care professional to answer live requests from customers.

To be a useful tool, patient material should at a minimum cover all of the following criteria:

- ➢ What benefits and problems to expect
- ➢ How, when, and for how long to take the medicine
- ➢ What treatments to avoid because of interactions with the new medication
- ➢ What to do if a dose is forgotten
- ➢ What to do if problems arise
- ➢ What kinds of problem to report immediately to a health care provider

The PEACEFUL elements are not all created equal; the discussion with the field representative will vary depending on the drug. For example, when a me-too drug (one that is structurally very similar to already approved drugs [same class], with only minor differences) is being evaluated, the safety, ease of use, and cost are most important. Still, the tool is useful to maximize the practitioner's interaction with the field representative and to focus attention on the information needed to keep a practice up to date.

Another useful tool for evaluating new drugs is the "drug dossier" prepared by the pharmaceutical company according to the Academy of Managed Care Pharmacy (AMCP) guidelines. AMCP developed several years ago a Format for Formulary Submissions (by industry) to improve the quality, scope, and relevance of information available to decision makers (http://www.amcp.org/data/nav_content/formatv20.pdf). This tool requires pharmaceutical companies to construct dossiers that provide critically appraised clinical and economic evidence supporting the efficacy and safety of the new drug. Each dossier contains the following sections: product information, supporting clinical and economic information, an impact economic model (to predict the economic consequences of formulary changes), clinical value, and overall cost.

For practitioners just wanting to stay updated, the dossiers provide more than the basic information because they are usually quite comprehensive—and sometimes lengthy. But they greatly reduce the time spent by a pharmacy and therapeutics committee member in searching for and recording the evidence needed to reach a formulary decision.

The Bottom Line

➤ Consider subscribing to an evidence-based subscription abstraction service.
➤ Invest in bibliographic management software to organize your information resources.
➤ Be selective in your information resources.
➤ Take control and focus on your information needs during pharmaceutical field representative visits.

References

1. Fact sheet: PubMed: Medline retrieval on the World Wide Web. Available at: http://www.nlm.nih.gov/pubs/factsheets/pubmed.html. Accessed November 28, 2006.

APPENDIX 8–A
PEACEFUL: APPRAISAL TOOL FOR A FOCUSED, COMPREHENSIVE INTERACTION WITH PHARMACEUTICAL FIELD REPRESENTATIVES

PEACEFUL	Comments
P̲atient's profile	
What is the FDA-approved indication?	Indication:
Who should receive it?	Age:
	Gender:
	Length of therapy:
Who should not receive it?	Caution/warnings:
Known drug interactions?	Contraindications:
E̲fficacy*	Outcomes:
Compared with placebo?	
Compared with gold standard?	
A̲vailability	
Hospital formulary?	
Health plans?	
Medicare/Medicaid?	
Included in other institutions' algorithms?†	

PEACEFUL	Comments
Cost[‡] Per treatment? Per unit? Indirect costs (laboratory tests, preparation time, etc.)?	
Ease of use More convenient than gold standard? Must be given with food? Requires special monitoring (CBC, LFTs, etc.)? Must be infused at a particular rate? Compatible with most common diluents?	
Formulations Available in different formulations (PO, syrup, SC, IV, IVBP, multidose vials, pens, etc.)?	
Unwanted side effects Minor side effects? Tolerability issues? Percent withdrawal due to side effects? Major side effects? Life-threatening side effects? Tolerability and major adverse event profile compared with gold standard therapy?	
Lay educational material Educational material for patients such as videos, starter kit, brochures, other patient tools available? Patient support programs (toll-free telephone number) available? Consumer Web sites available?	

CBC = Complete blood cell count; LFT = liver function test; PO = by mouth; SC = subcutaneous; IV = intravenous; IVBP = intravenously using pump.

* Request to see published evidence from peer-reviewed journals, an AMCP format drug dossier created according to the Academy of Managed Care Pharmacy format if available, and a review article published in a peer-reviewed journal.
† Request other institution's algorithm if possible.
‡ Request a published cost analysis if available.

INDEX

Page numbers followed by "t" denote tables; those followed by "f" denote figures